Sprinkled Clean

Small-Group Curriculum

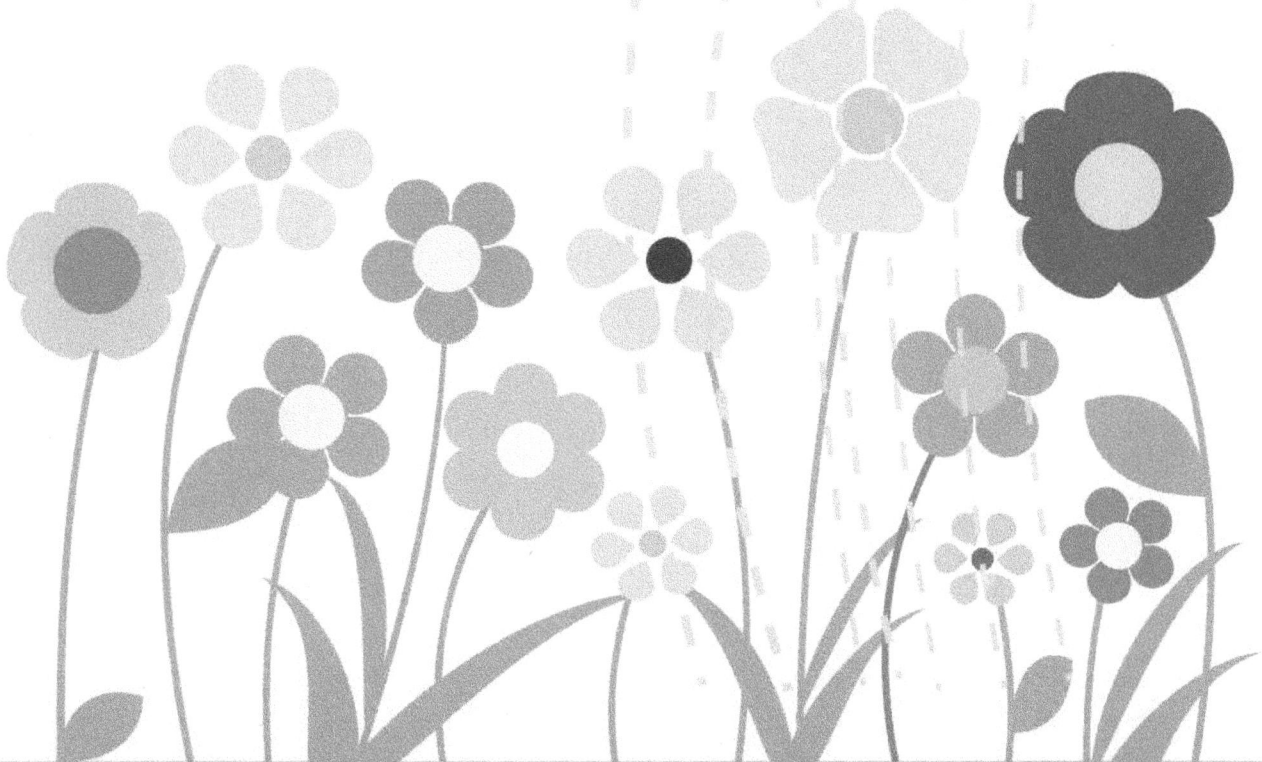

I0225371

Judi Ulrey

Sprinkled Clean

Halig Press is the self-publishing division of Fitness Consulting, a sole proprietorship promoting health and fitness since 1985.Holy Health Club (HolyHealthClub.com) and Live Well by Grace (LiveWellbyGrace.com) are subsidiaries thereof.

Copyright 2023 by Judi Ulrey

ISBN 978-0-9668042-2-5 Print
ISBN 978-0-9668042-5-6 Ebook

Unless otherwise identified, all Scripture quotations in this publication are taken from the English Standard Version (ESV), copyright 2001 by Crossway Bibles, a division of Good News Publishers.

To all those who claim Jesus Christ as Lord and Savior.

May your hearts be sprinkled with clean water,

by His grace, for His glory.

Contents

Insights by Grace sprinkled throughout are generously contributed by . . . Grace.
You can find her at http://www.LiveWellbyGrace.com

Then will I sprinkle clean water upon you, and ye shall be clean: from all your filthiness, and from all your idols, will I cleanse you.

EZEKIEL 36:25 (KJV)

Preface

I was horrified. Mom was screaming at the drugstore pharmacist, and I was cowering amongst the cold remedies lest I be associated with her.

Both my brother and sister are quick to anger. Me makes three. Seems the raging gene got passed down from one generation to another.

The late, great Jerry Bridges wrote a book entitled *Respectable Sins*, and anger is one of them. (NavPress 2007, 2010) He also addresses pride, selfishness, jealousy, and discontent, all of which the Church has been prone to ignore. We're only human, right? But after not one but two rounds of counseling, it became clear to me that my tempestuous spirit and potty mouth not only didn't glorify God, they were downright disobedience.

After three decades of developing employee wellness campaigns, I was disheartened by the general lack of permanent lifestyle change. Oh sure, folks would walk for a while to earn a cool t-shirt, then would slowly revert back to their sedentary ways. My own failure in tempering my tantrums elevated my empathy for those who struggle with food and exercise discipline. Nike prods, "Just do it," but if that wasn't working for me and my mouth, why would willpower be the answer to another's stronghold? I slowly began to understand that without spiritual transformation by the power of the Holy Spirit, I would forever battle with my ire; likewise for those who have been disappointed by diets.

Originally, I thought I was writing a Christian fitness book with scripture sprinkled in. To my surprise it became a Bible-laden work with fitness tips included. But Proverbs 16:9 is clear: *The heart of man plans his way, but the Lord establishes his steps.* He prodded me to look yet again at my own failings, revealing that your struggle with over-eating and under-moving is no different than my struggle with judgment and pride, the source of my anger. I pray my journey toward transformation will kindle yours.

Sprinkled Clean offers encouragement and hope for Christians who aspire to eat more healthfully, move more regularly, and pray more earnestly. If you accept that without Him you can do nothing – NO thing – this workbook is for you. You are done with diets. You acknowledge you abhor exercise. You eat what's easy and/or momentarily satisfying but are seeing the side effects. And finally, it's for those who are willing to admit they need support. You're ready to both garner and give encouragement "to stir one another up to love and good deeds." The heart is healed through helping.

Sincere thanks to my dear sister Tricia, who walked with me faithfully prior to and through the completion of *Sprinkled Clean*. As God transformed my stony heart, she corrected my pitiful punctuation.

The Church is highly committed to supporting one another in our spiritual and emotional growth, but discussing physical apathy seems taboo. Well, I was never much good at following the rules, so let's start talking.

Prayerfully submitted,

Judi Ulrey

Introduction

God can change you.

Do you believe that? Do you *really* believe that?

Can God truly transform you, including those pesky, persistent, unhealthy habits?

Like all of us, you may have more than one "personality quirk" that could use some revamping. As you will read, mine was impatience and anger. After three decades of health promotion, this workbook was written for those who struggle with physical discipline. You want to be more consistent with your exercise, but you're frenetically busy. Your menu needs a makeover, but shopping and cooking are inconvenient. And truth be told, you're a little ambivalent about this tending your temple business. I mean really, don't you have enough on your plate? (Pun intended.) ☺

God *can* change you.

The "I can't do this" mentality is the old you. 2 Corinthians 5:17 tells us *the old has passed away, behold, the new has come.* That means unhealthy and unhelpful thoughts, attitudes, and habits, are all remnants of your old self. "But," you say, "I've tried and I can't." Here's the good news: God can. He will give you a new heart with new affections. All things – even physical transformation – are possible through Christ (Philippians 4:13).

As you consider making different, sometimes uncomfortable, choices, invite someone who also struggles to join you. According to the US Center for Disease Control, many Americans could use some encouragement. The paragraph below comes from their website https://www.cdc.gov/diabetes/prevention/prediabetes-type2/index.html:

"More than 84 million US adults—that's 1 in 3—have prediabetes. With prediabetes, blood sugar is higher than normal but not high enough yet to be diagnosed as diabetes. People with prediabetes are at high risk for type 2 diabetes (the most common type), heart disease, and stroke.

In the last 20 years, the number of adults diagnosed with diabetes has more than tripled as the US population has aged and become more overweight. Now more than 30 million Americans have diabetes, which increases their risk for a long list of serious health problems, including:

- Heart attack
- Stroke

- Blindness
- Kidney failure
- Loss of toes, feet, or legs"

In case statistics don't move you, let's make this a bit more personal. For every hundred members of your church, over thirty are at high risk of devastating health challenges. Think about it. Who sits in your pew week after week? Of those fifteen people, five are walking toward a life-altering health event. Invite them on this journey with you, then grab their hands and slowly change course together.

God can change the church.

Have you ever noticed how many prayer requests related to ill-health are uplifted, week-after-week, in churches across America? Joe's heart attack. Mary, who's been overweight most of her life, fell and broke her hip. The Miller boy, "big" for his age, has just been diagnosed with what used to be called "adult onset" diabetes. The life of the Body is impacted by the health (or lack thereof) of our bodies. Going out into all the world requires physical strength and verve.

Paul didn't mince words with the Corinthian church. Though they were guilty of sexual immorality, the message remains. *Or do you not know that your body is a temple of the Holy Spirit within you, whom you have from God? You are not your own, for you were bought with a price. So glorify God in your body* (1 Corinthians 6:19-20).

According to the Cleveland Clinic, tending our temple includes embracing healthy habits: "Poor lifestyle choices, such as smoking, overuse of alcohol, poor diet, lack of physical activity, and inadequate relief of chronic stress are key contributors in the development and progression of preventable chronic diseases, including obesity, type 2 diabetes mellitus, hypertension, cardiovascular disease and several types of cancer." [https://my.clevelandclinic.org/health/transcripts/1444_lifestyle-choices-root-causes-of-chronic-diseases] But a sobering study by Duke School of Divinity, quoted by Scott Stoll, MD in his provocative book, *Alive!** found Christians are slacking in our tending:

- 70% of Americans are overweight or obese.
- 76% of evangelical Christians are overweight or obese.
- 76% of evangelical pastors are overweight or obese

---

* *Alive!* By Scott Stoll, MD, Creative Enterprises Studio, 2011

Dr. Stoll says, "As Christians begin to lose their health, they become focused on their own lives, pain, diseases, and sufferings, which leaves them less able to focus on the needs around them. The ability to rise up and go forth, to see and meet the needs around us is greatly diminished, and the living, active church slowly dies from within."

Wow. Painful truth.

But God can change the Church.

I am intrigued by Moses' words in Exodus 33:16: *For how shall it be known that I have found favor in your sight, I and your people? Is it not in your going with us, so that we are distinct, I and your people, from every other people on the face of the earth?* When we look at the fitness statistics above, are Christians *physically* distinct? Is it clear we have favor in God's sight to overcome the strongholds of temptation and addiction? If not, why not?

God's Word is rife with the call to Christian service, but we all need to be regularly reminded. Muse on the passages below:

In all things I have shown you that by working hard in this way we must help the weak and remember the words of the Lord Jesus, how he himself said, "It is more blessed to give than to receive (Acts 20:35).

⁹And let us not grow weary of doing good, for in due season we will reap, if we do not give up. ¹⁰So then, as we have opportunity, let us do good to everyone, and especially to those who are of the household of faith (Galatians 6:9-10).

Next, refresh your memory on James' message on faith and works in James 2:14-24.

Then there was the good Samaritan . . .

Do you pray for your eyes to be opened for opportunities to serve?

Jesus said to his followers, *I have come that you might have life, and have it abundantly* (John 10:10). Abundant means full, bountiful, exuberant, rich. Are Christians experiencing God's bountiful, rich, abundant life to the fullest? Or are we less able to serve due to our own suffering, as Dr. Stoll suggests?

The good news is Christians can cling to the Good News. We have been re-created in Christ. Though we tend toward passions of the flesh, by the renewing of our minds and surrender to the Spirit we can overcome the lures of this world and live fully and healthfully.

God can change the Church.

What if we earnestly petitioned Him to help us in our physical as well as spiritual disciplines? *The effectual fervent prayer of a righteous man availeth much* (James 5:16, KJV). As we gather in small groups across the country, "doing life together" as the family of God, shall we deliberately arouse our health as well as our hearts? Hebrews 10:24-25 says, *And let us consider how to stir up one another to love and good works, not neglecting to meet together, as is the habit of some, but encouraging one another, and all the more as you see the Day drawing near.* What if we regularly met together to walk? Or inspired one another to eat healthfully? When you uplift another, you arise too.

The Gospel can change the world.

Christ-followers are exceedingly charitable. From building hospitals and schools, to offering financial assistance and regularly lending a helping hand, the Church cares. What if in addition to building hospitals, we also worked to keep folks out of them.

According to the Boston Medical Center's website, "45 million Americans go on a diet every year, spending $33 billion on weight loss products. Yet, nearly two-thirds of Americans are overweight or obese. Obesity is a chronic disease that requires lifelong treatment and medical care." (https://www.bmc.org/nutrition-and-weight-management/weight-management) Let's translate that: 60% of Americans are spending loads of dough for weight-loss products and programs that don't work. They're buying into "lifelong treatment and medical care." Something's amok here. If the Church could offer them truths that truly transformed them, would they? Should they? Of course! The truth is diets based on tips and tricks and willpower are futile, but complete surrender and reliance on God Almighty is transformational. He can give us a new heart with new affections. All things – even physical transformation – are possible through Christ. The $33 billion weight loss programs don't work because they're missing the all-important, solely sanctifying ingredient: Jesus.

The Gospel can change the world.

Evangelism is one of our callings as Christians. *Go into all the world and preach the gospel* (Mark 16:15). God's good news is not just for spiritual healing, but physical too. Let me be clear: I'm not saying anyone and everyone will be cured of cancer, heart disease, you name the malady. But what I *am* saying is God is bigger than your flesh. Just ask the woman who was bleeding non-stop for twelve years. *If I touch even His garments, I will be made well* (Mark 5:28). She did, and she was. As the Church not only acknowledges her own need for the Healer, but also opens its doors to outsiders, showing non-believers how they can be transformed through Christ, lives will change, both today and eternally. And what about that person who experiences physical renewal through the Spirit? Like the woman at the well, she's going to tell all her friends, and churches will be filled with newcomers who have seen the world's ways don't work.

The Gospel can change the world.

As Christians overcome the temptations of the flesh, and encourage the world to surrender to the Spirit too, how might that impact society? What if obesity, heart disease, and stroke were cut in half? What if adult-onset diabetes, especially in affected children, began to "mysteriously" decline? Can you imagine if the trending news ten years from now is a study by the Robert Wood Johnson Foundation, reporting that health statistics, specifically within the Christian community, have been dramatically improving, reducing the overall cost of healthcare? We would enlarge our testimony – a story to give God glory.

This workbook doesn't recommend a diet. Though I'll propose several healthy habits in The Lab (which you undoubtedly could recite by rote), this isn't about boycotting bread or mastering the latest fitness moves. It's about Jesus' ability to change your life; God going with you so you are distinct. God's grace is the obvious and all-important missing ingredient in most food and fitness programs. For without Him you can do nothing. NO thing. Period. But with God *all* things are possible.

Every child of God is unique. The combination of our life experiences, circumstances, relationships, and beliefs lead us to process life and its lessons differently. Yet there are a handful of universal spiritual and physical truths. My intention is to use the *spiritual* disciplines to provide you vision and strength to tackle the *physical* disciplines. True transformation requires reflection and prayer. It is imperative that each week you not just think about the proffered questions but take the time to write out your answers. Print the pages and put pen in hand, or buy yourself a notebook or journal. Then when you and your friend and/or small group gather, you'll remember what the Spirit whispered to you. It will steer the conversation of thoughts, feelings, and epiphanies, in addition to determining how you can support each other in applying the Fitness Focus, or actions steps. Finally, your writings become an adjunct to your Prayer Journal, for transformation requires intercession.

Another big difference between *Sprinkled Clean* and other diet/weight loss books, including Christian publications, is it was specifically developed to be done in pairs or small groups. Ecclesiastes 4:12 is clear: *Though a man might prevail against one who is alone, two will withstand him – a threefold cord is not quickly broken.* We, the Church, are called to support, uplift, and encourage one another, and that includes making wise choices, especially when our cravings cry out otherwise.

But let's start at the beginning.

God's Gracious Gift

Consider the gift of the Gospel. God Almighty, maker of heaven and earth, all-powerful and all-knowing, desperately wants to have an intimate relationship with you. He yearns to share your good times and bad, your ups and downs. When you question your direction, He is quick to lead. He wants *...to strengthen you, to help you, to uphold you with my righteous right hand* (Isaiah 41:10).

But in your corrupt condition, He couldn't commune with you. From the moment you popped out of your mother's womb, your human DNA made you deplorable. You were *dead in trespasses and sins . . . following the course of this world . . . in the passions of your flesh* (Ephesians 2:1-3). You were stubborn, greedy, self-centered, and envious, not to mention fearful, doubt-full, and angry. Who'd want to hang out with you?

God would.

But God, being rich in mercy, because of the great love with which He loves us, even when we were dead in our trespasses, made us alive together with Christ – by grace you have been saved – and raised us up with Him and seated us with Him in the heavenly places in Christ Jesus (Ephesians 2:4-7). He sent His son Jesus, the Word, who was with God and was God, to pay the ransom for our failings. He died that we might have life. *By grace you have been saved by faith* (Ephesians 2:8). You didn't deserve grace, but it's who He is. *He is full of grace and truth* (John 1:14). Salvation by faith is a gift, *not* a kudo or reward (Ephesians 2:8). As you come to recognize your need for a Savior, you are moved by faith to acknowledge His holy sacrifice, humbly surrender your life, and let Him lead. You become united to Him; all that He is becomes yours. This is your regeneration, being brought from spiritual death to life. *If you confess with your mouth that Jesus is Lord and believe in your heart that God raised Him from the dead, you will be saved* (Romans 10:9). The strength, help, and hand-holding promised in Isaiah 41:10 is obtained solely through faith. Believing before seeing. Trusting that His thoughts are higher than yours, and that He is your ever-present help in time of need.

And that "time of need" includes overcoming destructive desires. Whether it's over-spending, greed, lust, gluttony, love of comfort, complacency, or over-eating when your heart hurts, Jesus says, "_____ (insert your name), I died for that. I conquered death. I defeated the flesh, and so you can live free from your disordered desires."

Does that make you crumble in gratitude? All those years you've struggled to "be good" in your own strength, now you can rely on grace alone, through Christ alone, for His name's sake. Did you catch that profound sentence two paragraphs north? You become united to Him; all that He is becomes yours. This is your regeneration, being brought from spiritual death to life. Finally, you can quit trying and start trusting. You can walk in faith as a new creation, claiming your new self. Conquering the desires of the flesh of any kind can only be Gospel-driven. Confess that you can't; believe that He can. Die to your deceitful desires and step into the abundant life He's called you to. *I can do all things through Christ who strengthens me*, said Paul to the Philippians (4:13). The Source of physical transformation is identical to the spiritual: in Christ alone, through faith alone, in His grace, by His power, for His glory. Period. Diets be damned. (Ooooppss, can I say that?)

As you progress on this trek toward transformation, remember God's helping you. Amidst the many hurdles, recognize Who's upholding you. Ingest Isaiah 41:10 as your moment-by-moment mantra. Rely on His strength, His help, His righteous right hand.

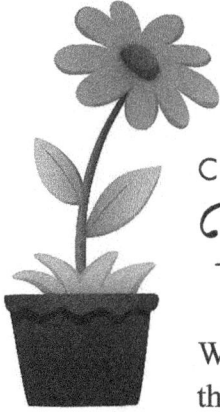

CHAPTER 1
Re-Define Your Why

What brings you here? What prompted you and your pal to commit to this process?

Every January 2nd, scores of Americans re-commit to "getting into shape." They overhaul their menus, fast from favorite foods, dust off their tennies and hit the pavement. But why are most resolutions aborted by Valentines Day? We need to rethink our motives.

For since the creation of the world God's invisible qualities – His eternal power and divine nature – have been clearly seen, being understood from what has been made, so that people are without excuse (Romans 1:20).

One of the many ways God reveals his glory is through creation. Did you know it was recently discovered that there are actually hundreds of galaxies, and that we, the Milky Way residents, may not be the center of the universe? As incomprehensible as the concept of other moons, stars, and planets in our solar system is, try grasping multiple galactic communities. Clearly, we can't. But one way we can attempt to fathom the glory and goodness of God is to consider our own bodies. Take a moment to muse:

Your heart beats 60-80 times every minute, completely independent of your efforts. It pumps blood throughout an inconceivably intricate network of pipes, day in and day out, carrying oxygen to your organs, cells, muscles, and brain. Imagine if you laid an adult's blood vessels end-to-end, including arteries, veins and capillaries, they would extend nearly 100,000 miles. (The Franklin Institute, https://www.fi.edu/heart/blood-vessels) We *cannot* imagine. Did you know a drop of blood contains 250 million cells? It's baffling. Have you ever considered your lungs? Oxygen transport on auto-pilot. Do you know you have six different muscles that control the movement in your eyes? Our body's complexity is truly beyond comprehension.

How do the above facts impact your thoughts about God?

_____

_____

Pondering the wonder of the Almighty is surely worthy of regular meditation. God's glory is humbling. Somewhat overwhelming. Contrite worship is our only reasonable response. We identify with the words of the Psalmist who said, *What is man, that You are mindful of him, and the son of man that you care for him?* (Psalm 8:4). But He did. And He does.

Personal motivation determines sustainability. Perceived benefits create consistency.

- You go to work because you're fond of the paycheck.
- You endure the commute because you like where you live.
- You put on make-up and coif your hair because it makes you feel pretty.

What is your motivation for caring for your body? Is it significant enough to keep you committed?

_____

_____

Let's look at God's guidance in the physical realm, starting with 1 Corinthians 6:19-20:

[19]Or do you not know that your body is a temple of the Holy Spirit within you, whom you have from God? You are not your own, [20]for you were bought with a price. So, glorify God in your body. This passage is a common go-to for those attempting to encourage the Body to care for their bodies, but unfortunately some hear it and spiral into shame. Remember, God is like a coach encouraging you, not berating you.

You are not your own. You have been bought with a price. So, glorify God in your body. How might you hear the Spirit whispering to you in this passage concerning your food and fitness?

_____

_____

Let's consider next our call to reflect Christ – to acknowledge and relish our Christ-likeness. Note any application to your food /fitness choices.

Therefore, if anyone is in Christ, he is a new creation. The old has passed away; behold, the new has come (2 Corinthians 5:17).

This one is a conundrum. It's clearly true, because it is God's holy Word. I don't know about you, but there are a *lot* of days when I feel like my old, selfish self is alive and well.

How can you claim this verse to support you in your new food/fitness journey?

_____

_____

Let's circle back to the twin verses in 1 Corinthians.

All things are lawful for me, but not all things are helpful. All things are lawful for me, but I will not be dominated by anything (1 Corinthians 6:12).

All things are lawful, but not all things are helpful. All things are lawful, but not all things build up (1 Corinthians 10:23).

Let's dissect.

[12]*All things are lawful for me, but not all things are helpful.* What an amazing God we serve! Consider the freedom He avails us in all things. Especially in America, we are free to worship, or not. At liberty to read the Word, or not. To care for our temple, or not. John 8:36 says, . . . *if the Son sets you free, you will be free indeed.* But though all things are lawful, Paul warns the Corinthians that not all things are helpful.

Are some foods more helpful than others? List 10 helpful foods and rate each one a 1-5 relative to how often you eat them. 1 = never, 2 = rarely, 3 = sometimes, 4 = regularly, 5 = often

_____   _____

_____   _____

_____   _____

_____   _____

_____   _____

Are there foods that are downright unhelpful? List a few and rate them on the scale above.

_____   _____

_____   _____

_____   _____

_____   _____

_____   _____

Is exercise helpful? List the reasons why or why not.

_____

_____

All things are lawful for me, but I will not be dominated by anything. The antithesis of freedom is slavery. Imprisonment. Captivity. Unfortunately, despite our freedom in Christ, we can become enslaved by things in the world. The lures of the flesh become all-consuming, overpowering our thoughts and actions. Be honest, does food generally, and certain foods specifically, tyrannize your thoughts? What does that look like?

List any foods you regularly consume, then afterwards regret.

_____

_____

Note any beliefs, fears, or excuses about embracing healthy habits that can sometimes derail you. Describe one of those instances.

_____

_____

All things are lawful, but not all things build up.

Building up connotes progress. Improvement. Synonyms include reinforce, expand, strengthen, boost, enhance. What behaviors build up?

_____

_____

Paul reminds the church in Acts 20 that *fierce wolves will come in among you, not sparing the flock* (Acts 20:29). He admonished them to stay in *the Word of His grace, which is able to build you up and to give you the inheritance among all those who are sanctified.* So clearly studying the scriptures build us up. He also tells the church in Thessalonica to *encourage one another and build on another up,* so Bible-based fellowship builds up.

Do your current food and fitness habits strengthen, boost, reinforce, and enhance your health? Why or why not?

_____

_____

According to the scripture, Christians have different inspiration for self-care than the world. Most folks want to lose weight to look better, feel better, and reduce risk of illness and injury. These are all valid aspirations, but Christ-followers have a unique perspective. The gift of the gospel explored in the introduction establishes a distinct foundation. When one considers God's love, revealed by Jesus' sacrifice, tending her temple becomes an act of gratitude and worship. And since He has promised to provide strength, help, and His righteous right hand, can you approach the process with confidence, and even enthusiasm? Explain.

_____

_____

The first question in the Westminster Catechism is, "What is the chief end of man?" Answer: "Man's chief end is to glorify God, and to enjoy Him forever." When you consider the statistics provided by Dr. Stoll in the introduction, that 76% of evangelical pastors and their flocks are overweight or obese, are we glorifying God with our bodies? Is glorifying God part of your Why? When the world sees a saint living victoriously over any tough issue, defeating the desires of the flesh through surrender to the Spirit, God is glorified. Note how/if that inspires you.

_____

_____

. . . *and to enjoy Him forever.* Are you often tired, achy, and/or physically restricted? Could you relish God and His gifts more vigorously if you had more energy? Describe what that would look like.

_____

_____

Then there is our call to service. Dr. Stoll says, "As Christians begin to lose their health, they become focused on their own lives, pain, diseases, and sufferings, which leaves them less able to focus on the needs around them. The ability to rise up and go forth, to see and meet the needs around us is greatly diminished, and the living, active church slowly dies from within." Has there ever been a time when your physical condition diminished your ability to serve? Describe here, and share with a friend.

_____

_____

How might you better minister to others if you were firing on all four cylinders?

_____

_____

Lack of perseverance is a common impediment to success, but in our own strength we inevitably falter. One of the many profound passages in the Bible is in John 15:5: *I am the vine; you are the branches. Whoever abides in me and I in him, he it is that bears much fruit, for apart from me you can do nothing.*

Don't you love how the punctuation proclaims the frank, definitive truth? Can you envision Jesus gathering his disciples for a moment of plainspoken instruction? "OK, gang, sit down. Let me make this really, really clear. I am the vine; you are the branches. I am the wind; you are the sailboat. I am the gas; you are the car. Got it? Without Me you're goin' nowhere."

Are you trying to improve your health through your own power? Do some truth-telling here as to what that looks like.

_____

_____

_____

God's grace is a gospel pillar. He did what we couldn't do, and gave what we didn't deserve. It calls us to let go of our self-sufficiency and admit our God-dependency. Accepting God's grace requires admitting our weakness, acknowledging our feelings are fickle, and trusting Him in all things.

That includes your body.

You can't. Jesus can. Abide in Him, and you can.

2 Thessalonians 1:11-12 may become a foundational verse in your temple tending process: [11]*To this end we always pray for you, that our God may make you worthy of his calling and may fulfill every resolve for good and every work of faith by his power,* [12]*so that the name of our Lord Jesus may be glorified in you, and you in him, according to the grace of our God and the Lord Jesus Christ.*

Are you stirred to surrender your self-sufficiency and declare your dependency on Christ? What if you saw your food and fitness trials and temptations as an opportunity to experience His power perfected in your weakness? Do some dittling about that. (I know, I know, dittle isn't currently a word, but it should be. Doodle's cousin.)

_____

_____

We have hopefully established that glorifying God, through transformation by grace, in His power alone, for His glory alone, is our true motivation for change. Each of you, however, also has legitimate personal reasons for improving your health. In addition to the spiritual benefits, what is your private, deep-down Why? Not to look good at the upcoming wedding or class reunion, but your heart-felt motive for improving your health. Are you concerned about a lifestyle-related disease? Is your ill-health impacting your relationships? Maybe you want to be a better role model for your kids. Write a letter to a famous personal trainer who is accepting one client pro bono. Why should it be you?

_____

_____

_____

_____

Let's review some of the possible reasons for committing to self-care:

- ▸ You want to do what's helpful.
- ▸ You don't want to be dominated by anything.
- ▸ Because God calls us to.
- ▸ Because your body is the temple of the Holy Spirit.
- ▸ You want to glorify God.
- ▸ You want to fully enjoy God.
- ▸ You want to fully serve God.
- ▸ You want to be fully dependent on Him.
- ▸ You want to be a role model for your kids, to have more energy for the grandkids, to have a more active life . . . .

The Word brings hope. Romans 15:13 says, *May the God of hope fill you with all joy and peace in believing, so that by the power of the Holy Spirit you may abound in hope.*

Now that you're clear your hope is in God's strength and not yours, calling you to cease striving and *know* that He – the Vine – is God, describe your physical condition and lifestyle at the age of 80. Be specific. Provide nitty gritty details. i.e. Who will be attending your soirée in celebration of your 8th decade? Where will it be, what will you eat, and how will you honor the occasion?

_____

_____

_____

When you get to the place of better tending your temple, what exactly are you doing, eating, and feeling? How is your life different, for better or worse?

_____

_____

_____

Fitness Focus:

This should be a simple exercise because you've already done the work. Using your answers to the earlier questions, write in one place why you want to commit – *permanently* commit – to physical care. What is your deep-down, grace-based, Why?

_____

_____

_____

Next, consider your typical food list. Are there foods that are lawful, but unhelpful to you? Start to take note. We'll deal with them later.

Living, Heart-piercing Words

There are a handful of verses worth packing for your coming excursion. (Well, there are more than a handful.) Meditate on these regularly. After each, use the probing questions to ponder how the passage relates to your journey toward a healthier lifestyle.

. . . remembering you in my prayers that the God of our Lord Jesus Christ, The Father of glory, may give you the Spirit of wisdom and of revelation in the knowledge of Him, having the eyes of your hearts enlightened, that you may know what is the hope to which He has called you, what are the riches of His glorious inheritance in the saints and what is the immeasurable greatness of His power toward us who believe, according to the working of His great might that He worked in Christ when He raised him from the dead (Ephesians 1:17-20).

Have you ever begun a food or fitness program by focusing on Jesus?

_____

What is the hope to which you believe He has called you in the physical realm?

_____

As a child of God, what inherited riches can assist you in your fitness journey?

_____

Has His power historically impacted your process? Explain.

_____

[14]For all who are led by the Spirit of God are sons of God. [15]For you did not receive the spirit of slavery to fall back into fear, but you have received the Spirit of adoption as sons, by whom we cry, "Abba! Father!" [16]The Spirit himself bears witness with our spirit that we are children of God, [17]and if children, then heirs—heirs of God and fellow heirs with Christ, provided we suffer with him in order that we may also be glorified with him (Romans 8:14-17).

Be honest. Do you harbor any fear over starting a food/fitness program, again? Talk to the One who *chose you,* here:

_____

_____

_____

Can you envision your life being a testimony to God's faithfulness and transformative power when you are finally free from physical bondage? Jot your thoughts.

_____

_____

_____

Do you see the difference between relying on willpower vs. God fulfilling every resolve for good? Envision yourself facing one of your familiar places of temptation. Talk yourself out of the corner through self-will. Then replay the scene, instead seeing yourself praying: "Lord, according to Your grace, make me worthy of Your calling. Fulfill my resolve for good choices. Help me. May you be glorified." How does this approach impact your strategy and confidence?

_____

_____

_____

My prayer for you: *May mercy, peace, and love be multiplied to you* (Jude 2).

Ready to dive in? Let me begin by sharing some of my own story.

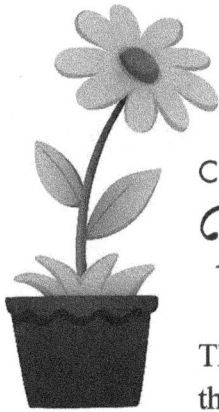

CHAPTER 2
Dear Abby, I'm Crabby

The following is a true story. The names have not been changed to protect the guilty.

Wednesday, September 8, 2010. 6:30 a.m.

With a suitcase, a computer (large in those days), and a small Dooney and Bourke shoulder bag, I knew I was over the carry-on limit, but imagined the baggage police wouldn't start growling this early in the morning.

"You'll need to put that purse inside your bag," the Frontier agent said as she scanned my ticket. Since I'd carried the same purse on four different flights on two different airlines within the previous ten days, I assumed the mandate scripted, but less-than-serious. I scowled and headed into the jetway.

Upon entering the plane, I was told again by one of the welcome crew to pack the 8" purse. I did, admittedly muttering something about pettiness, at which point she began reciting FAA rules. "Shut up! Just let me get to my seat," my brain retaliated. All I wanted was to be left alone to eat my bagel in peace. (Bagel? Definitely a decade ago . . .)

After settling in, computer tucked under my front neighbor's seat and my purse safely on the floor behind my feet, another attendant came by and directed me to stash the purse with the computer. After I did, visibly begrudgingly, she continued to hover, saying I also needed to store the white paper breakfast bag.

At what point do "safety measures" become harassment?

I shoved my bagel under the seat and glared, "Are you happy?" Ms. Attendant leaned within two inches of my face and said "I'm tired of your attitude. FAA is on board and you could be asked to leave." Wow. Who knew a bagel and a bag could raise such ire. I buried in my book, trying to survive the hostile environment. The plane pulled out. I was finally on my way.

You might imagine my shock when the captain announced soon thereafter that they would be pulling back to the gate to let a passenger off. The minute we stopped, four armed police officers boarded the plane, came directly to my seat and asked me to gather my belongings and follow them. Really? I'm kicked off a flight for being cranky? Within ten minutes a tall, gently graying man arrived at the gate and showed me his badge. "Hello. My name is Charles McGregor. I'm with Homeland Security . . . "

What's your story?

Describe a time when a failure to eat well or exercise stemmed from demanding your own way.

_____

_____

Do you find yourself refusing to follow the rules, that ironically, you actually set for yourself? Talk to yourself about that.

_____

_____

When was the last time you snuck in a snack, hoping the food police weren't watching? What were your thoughts/feelings afterwards?

_____

_____

Angry at God

Know this, my beloved brothers, let every person be quick to hear, slow to speak, slow to anger (James 1:19).

Testy. Explosive. Don't cross her. These are a sampling of words and phrases friends and acquaintances might have used to describe me. Unfortunately, irritability wasn't one of the Fruit of the Spirit, and those that did make the list seemed a fantasy for me. Patience? Kindness? Don't count on it with this one.

But like many who start a diet on January 2nd, it was always a should. I should try harder to manage my mouth – accept others' failings and foibles – be slower to judge. If I could only remember to stop and take some deep breaths, my anger would magically dissipate, right?

Wrong.

In reflecting back on that fateful flight (that I missed . . .) in the fall of 2010, anger had accomplices. Additional descriptors would include snitty, antagonistic, and prideful. "Who are you to tell me what to do," my insolence implied. My insistence on openly carrying my bag was more important than following "their" rules. In hindsight a decade past, I'm befuddled and embarrassed by my behavior. There's no question the small shoulder bag would have *easily* fit into my carry-on. It was unadulterated, bratty belligerence.

They say most need to hit bottom before they are willing to admit they have a problem and seek help. My unscheduled meeting with Homeland Security was my bottom, and my subsequent prod to honestly address my anger issues. Living at the time in a little mountain town in southern California, I was surprised and encouraged to find a Celebrate Recovery group. "Hi, my name is Judi, and if I don't get my way, I spit venom."

The probing questions excavated a treasure trove of ancient hurts and scars, providing insights, though not excuses. But a mid-March 2011 letter to my pastor and his wife launched my sanctification process to the next phase. To avoid undue rambling, the gist of my message was "God is untrustworthy and unloving because He hasn't sufficiently provided for me financially." They recommended I talk to a local Christian counselor named Tricia. "She will be able to walk you Biblically through your questions and doubts."

That was the beginning of a journey that continues to slowly wind up the mountain, even today.

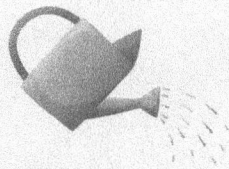

You will seek me and find me, when you seek me with all your heart (Jeremiah 29:13).

They say (Who are "they" anyway?), "follow your dreams and the money will follow." Well, I am living proof "they" can be sorely mistaken.

For reasons to be revealed, I was an avid bike rider as a kid. I'd spend hours and hours on my yellow Schwinn Le Tour, roaming rural byways, escaping chaos at home. Post college, after completing a term paper on corporate wellness, I was convinced I'd found the perfect combination of my business degree and fitness passion. I stuffed every nook and cranny of my silver Honda Civic with all my worldly possessions and drove myself to southern California. My plan was to attend Cal Poly San Luis Obispo, get a Master's degree in Exercise Physiology, and work for a big company as their Corporate Wellness Manager. While waiting the year to establish residency, I found a small company who provided individual fitness testing and food and exercise consulting. They offered me hands-on training in much of the Cal Poly curriculum. What did I have to lose?

To summarize a year into a paragraph, under their tutelage I mastered hydrostatic (underwater) weighing, cardiovascular fitness testing, basic nutrition, and exercise prescription. I was "dunking" clients, assessing their lean-to-fat weight ratio based on their personal goals, and fine-tuning their fitness program. I was a happy camper. But within six months I discovered I was sailing on a sinking ship; they were headed for bankruptcy. After working the numbers all July 4th weekend, I made them an offer to buy their struggling business, and on September 1, 1985, I became an entrepreneur. Recollecting my term paper, I soon launched what became a three-decades long career in corporate wellness.

I followed my passion, but the money rarely followed. As the economy rose and fell, so did companies' already tepid commitment to promoting employee health. During my entire working career, I would have been considered a low-income earner.

Given that background, below are some excerpts from that letter to my pastor in early 2011:

> I have lately been processing my deep-seated fear, especially about money, and the subsequent anger that arises. This morning it became clear that that fear comes, in part, from perceiving God as unpredictable and not particularly loving . . . I think a love indicator is being trustworthy. If you love, you tell the truth. I may not always like what you say, but I know I can trust your words to be true.

> The gospels say *Ask and you shall receive. Ask whatever you wish and it shall be done for you.* Well, that's simply not true. I don't have a problem with not getting everything I ask for; I simply wish the Word was true. "Ask whatever you wish and if I feel like it, it shall be done for you," would be more accurately stated. Setting me up to ask and believe before I see, then not provide, feels very deceitful.

So, to believe that God loves me unconditionally requires that I turn my brain off to reality. He loves me, but He may or may not protect me from harm. I'm always in Divine Boot Camp. "Endure this and prove you still trust me!" He loves me, and has told me to ask and believe and keep knocking, but He'll provide (or not...) in His own good time. Waiting is another Boot Camp lesson. He loves me unconditionally, but woe to me if I quit bowing to Him.

Can you say raw and wrenching? I was ready to be real. I took the pastor's recommendation to speak to Tricia, who could help me "answer my questions." I wanted answers, so I picked up the phone and made my first appointment. She remembers clearly, "You came in shaking your fist at God." By that time, I had been in business for sixteen years, and still had a pauper's income. I was angry.

After all the introductory pleasantries, I plunged into my history and heartache. Getting booted off an airplane. My tendency to trigger. Constant lack of cash flow. "I love God, but . . . am tired of being in Boot Camp."

Tricia doesn't mince words. "God sent His Son to die on your behalf. If He did nothing else, ever, He has done more than you deserve."

I remember my chest tightening and tears trickling. I honestly and earnestly loved God. I understood the cost of Calvary. She handed me a tissue. The silence welcomed His Spirit. Tricia, I'm sure, was praying.

"You're right," I finally whispered. "But . . ." How should I say it? Do my struggles have no merit? Were her words just another way of saying, "Suck it up and get over it"?

Finally, my feelings fell out. "Why is He so mean? He says, 'Ask and ye shall receive,' and I've asked and asked and asked and waited and waited and waited, and still He doesn't provide enough for me to pay my bills. What about that parable about a man who works is worthy of a fair wage?"

"Let's back up a few steps," she calmly suggested. "Let's revisit the airplane incident. Tell me about your refusal to put the purse in your suitcase."

"I don't know," I replied, my eyes slipping toward the small stain on the carpet. "It just seems so stupid."

"But it's the airline's rule, and you were riding on their aircraft."

I looked right at her. "But what's the big deal? Yes, I should have stashed the bag. But that woman didn't need to get in my face."

"It was their third request." Tricia is always annoyingly composed.

Whose side is she on? And what does this have to do with God going AWOL on giving me a little financial favor?

"Why did you make it a big deal," Tricia asked in her straightforward, yet cool and collected way.

Dang, she wasn't going to let up.

"I hate stupid rules, . . . and stupid people telling me what to do."

"That sounds a lot like pride to me."

Silence fell again.

Job's (Judi's . . .) Pride

Will you even put me in the wrong? Will you condemn me that you may be in the right? (God to Job, 40:8).

Job's story confounded me. Right out of the box, the writer describes him as *blameless and upright, one who feared God and turned away from evil* (Job 1:1). How could a loving God allow Satan to emasculate one of His righteous, God-fearing sons?

Satan was convinced he could derail him, so God said, "Go ahead. Try. Just don't take his life." What about His promise to protect His people? The story fueled my distrust. I decided to reread it, seeking truth from God's perspective. "Lord, open the eyes of my heart."

Job's Story:

Satan doesn't waste any time, peppering Job with traumatic afflictions. First his property, then his family, and finally, his health. You can understand Job's devastation and confusion. Why would his Father allow this? By enumerating his good deeds in chapter 29, it's clear he considered himself as a decent guy. Helper of the weak. Provider to the poor. Counselor to the inexperienced. Definitely Elder material. He feels abandoned by the One who assured him He'd never leave nor forsake him. *I cry to you for help and you do not answer me; I stand, and you only look at me. You have turned cruel to me; with the might of your hand you persecute me* (Job 30:20-21). *Is not calamity for the unrighteous, and disaster for the workers of iniquity? Does not he see my ways and number all my steps?* (Job 31:3-4).

Sounds like my letter to my pastor, doesn't it?

How about you? Have you ever felt abandoned by your Father? Stuff keeps happening and you cry out, "Where are you, God? Why are you not hearing my cry?" Do you spin on your heels and shun Him, as I did? Take a moment to write down your thoughts and feelings when God feels far away.

Job's three besties are happy to offer inane insights. Eliphaz reminds Job that God is good to His faithful followers, so he must have messed up somewhere. "Repent and get back in God's good grace." Bildad is more brutal. He contends Job's kids were sinners who deserved to die, and if Job didn't repent, he'd be heading to heaven right behind them. Finally, Zophar jumps in, reminding Job the wicked only prevail for a short time before God gives them their just reward. How would you like to have these guys as friends?

Then some young buck by the name of Elihu walks on to the stage, insisting they're all wrong. "Sit down, fellas. I have a word for you from God."

Why do you contend against Him, saying, 'He will answer none of man's words' (Job 33:13).

"God did answer you, Job," Elihu argues. "He communicates by two means: in dreams and *through affliction.*"

This interpretation is staggering. Stand up for a minute, roll your shoulders, take some long, deep breaths, grab your Bible and read Job 33:19-30.

My stomach felt queasy after reading this passage. My brain swirling. I sheepishly peeked back over my shoulder at God, fists slowly unfurling. He was talking to me.

 "Man is also rebuked with pain on his bed . . . How many nights, year after year, did I live with unfettered anxiety over my meager income?

He is merciful to him, and says, 'Deliver him from going down into the pit; I have found a ransom; . . . . Trust in Me, Judith, not your bank balance. Remember, *fear not, for I am with you. Be not dismayed, for I am your God. I will strengthen you. I will help you. I will uphold you with my righteous right hand* (Isaiah 41:10).

²⁶*then man prays to God, and He accepts* (forgives) *him; He sees his face with a shout of joy, and He restores to man his righteousness.* After rereading old journals, I understood this perfectly described my previous process. I would humbly repent. God graciously forgave. My heart was at peace. Then I would go into fear and start whining again.

²⁷*He sings before men and says: 'I sinned and perverted what was right, and it was not repaid to me.* "You have redemption through Jesus. If He does nothing more, He has done enough."

²⁸*He has redeemed my soul from going down into the pit, and my life shall look upon the light.'* Being angry at God is *not* a peaceful place. Even if circumstances don't change, my heart is much happier when I trust there's a reason for the hardship. (More on this later.)

²⁹*"Behold, God does all these things, twice, three times, with a man,* ³⁰*to bring back his soul from the pit, that he may be lighted with the light of life* (Job 33:29-30*).* We humans are slow learners. We keep getting tried because we keep forgetting. *God does all these things twice, three times . . .* Sanctification is a *S-L-O-W*, life-long, again-and-again, arduous process. No gold medals this side of the pearly gates.

John Piper offers a superb sermon on this passage, suggesting we see difficult days as a healing act from a surgeon's knife, vs. an executioners sword; a refining vs. consuming fire (https://www.desiringgod.org/messages/job-rebuked-in-suffering). God was purging pride from Job's heart . . . and mine.

The Cross

Rereading the book of Job gave me a new view. Without question, he was being pummeled by problems, but he was also prideful. "How could You do this to me, LORD, when I have been so faithful to you?" Let's go back to Job 33:27, and Tricia's words:

He sings before men and says: 'I sinned and perverted what was right, and it was not repaid to me.

"You have redemption through Jesus. If He does nothing more, He has done enough."

He had done enough.

Had I acknowledged that? Did I believe that? Had I genuinely, repentantly, contritely, acknowledged Jesus' sacrifice at Calvary?

Judi's Journal 6/26/11

"What's with all the blood and guts?" The anger inside was barely manageable. I'm supposed to trust and worship this God who subjects even His own son to brutal killing? I thought He was supposed to be so compassionate? Not seein' it.

I've come in for anger counseling. The rage is out of control. It pops up so quickly – so unexpectedly – and woe to the person on whom it is unleashed. And Tricia has the audacity to suggest it's because I have no gratitude for the cross. Really? I'm supposed to somehow feel good about a God who demands blood and guts? I just can't connect those dots . . .

When was the last time you contemplated the gift of Calvary? In your opinion, has God done enough for you, or do you continue to demand? Take a moment to write your thoughts to God.

_____

_____

_____

_____

_____

_____

_____

_____

_____

_____

_____

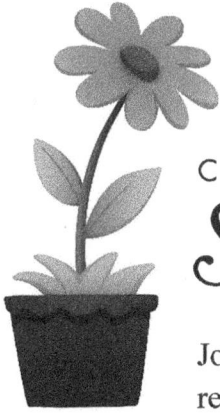

CHAPTER 3
Sinners All

Job's story and Tricia's counsel forced me to acknowledge my prideful rebellion. I wanted life on my terms. I'll make my own airplane rules, thank you. And I'll tell God what is an acceptable income that He might stay in my favor. In hindsight, it was heresy.

What say you? Are any of your imprudent food choices a by-product of prideful demands? Reflect here:

_____

_____

_____

_____

_____

_____

_____

_____

They say when you're in the market for a yellow, vintage Volkswagen, suddenly they pop up everywhere, so predictably, I happened upon a book entitled *The Bait of Satan*, by John Bevere. His premise is, offense is a trap Satan uses to hold Christians in bondage. A few excerpts:

"Pride causes you to view yourself as a victim . . . If we do not deal with an offense, it will produce more fruit of sin, such as bitterness, anger, and resentment . . . When we filter everything through past hurts, rejections, and experiences, we find it impossible to believe God. We cannot believe He means what He says. We doubt His goodness, and faithfulness since we judge Him by the standards set by man . . . We must be protected and safe at all costs." [*The Bait of Satan*, Charisma House]

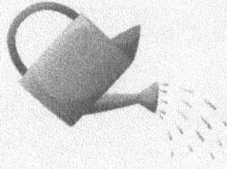

Riding Shotgun

"Get in the car, Judith, we're going for a drive." My mom was unusually intense.

"I can't. I have homework."

"You can finish your homework tonight. We have an errand to run." She was adamant.

"Where are we going?"

"In search of your father."

Dad was gone a lot in my growing up years. When he was home, he and Mom were usually going at it. He'd yell. She'd cry and lock herself in the bathroom. Then he'd yell at us, saying she was upset because we hadn't cleaned our rooms. So, when we went to look for him that memorable afternoon, I knew it wasn't to meet him at Cracker Barrel for supper.

I grew up in a rural Indianapolis suburb, abounding in corn fields and country roads. I wasn't old enough to drive, but knew exactly where we were that day, as our route followed that of my daily school bus ride. We hadn't driven far before Mom pulled on to a side road, stopped the car, got out and started taking pictures. What was Dad's car doing at that house? Why didn't we just go there and talk to him? My memory is blurry, but it seems like he quickly came out the front door and exchanged unwelcoming words with Mom across the field. But the next scene is forever etched in my brain: a woman slipped out from behind him, pointing a shotgun at Mom. "Get off my property," she shouted. Clearly, she wasn't going to invite us in for a cup of tea . . . Mom jumped back in the car, made me crouch down on the floor, and we tore off. Feeling cramped, I soon asked if I could get up, to which she replied, "No, your father's following us."

Well, isn't that good? Hadn't we gone to find him? Can't we discuss this over dinner?

"Listen carefully to me. I'm going to the Thompson's house. I'll pull in their driveway, and when I stop, you run in the front door. I'll come pick you up later."

"Why? Why can't I come home with you?"

"Your father and I need to talk. I'll call you when we're finished."

Again, the details don't come. I assume I hung out at the neighbor's awhile, and eventually made it home. I don't remember ever getting a debrief, nor whether my homework got finished.

Run for your life

Prey animals, like horses and deer, are always on alert, and quickly flee from danger, both real or imagined. Carey A. Williams, PhD, from Rutgers University, says, "The horse, a prey animal, depends on flight as its primary means of survival . . . Horses are one of the most perceptive of all domestic animals. Since they are a prey species, they must be able to detect predators. A stimulus unnoticed by humans is often cause for alarm for horses . . . Horses forgive, but they do not forget. They especially remember bad situations. This is why it is critical to make the horse's first training experience a positive one."

I'm not a psychologist, but seems to me prey people do the same.

Childhood memories imprint us. Month after month, year after year, lessons and lies become deeply ingrained. They can easily turn into the tracks we follow throughout life. Fear becomes who we are – the story we tell ourselves, and believe.

In a child's mind, when family isn't safe, everyone becomes a potential predator. Self-protection becomes our nature. Our internal drive. Our sole mission. Solitude, then, is the only safe place.

I learned early how to survive the drama on the home front. The woods behind our neighborhood was a regular retreat. Just three streets away, we were allowed to walk there. The towering trees protected me. Quiet enshrouded me like a soft, warm, blanket. Turmoil and tears couldn't find me. The path to peace was trod alone.

OK, so my childhood wasn't like the Cleaver's. (For you young bucks, search "Leave it to Beaver" on YouTube.) Does that give me the right to go through life with my fists poised to strike?

Your turn. What past hurts are impacting your decisions today? Do you make choices, either consciously or unconsciously, for self-protection? Is food your safe place? What thoughts go through your mind during these times?

_____

_____

_____

_____

There's a difference between a reason and an excuse. I get it that I have authority issues because my dad was a dictator. I understand how I came to believe that I'm only safe alone. It's a logical progression from survival to self-absorption. But that keeps the focus on me, and that never works out well.

Together, let's pray the King James version of Psalm 119:133: *Order my steps in Thy word; and let not any iniquity have dominion over me.*

Stumblers

Life happens. We all stumble – fall short. Even the apostle Paul said, *For I do not understand my own actions. For I do not do what I want, but I do the very thing I hate* (Romans 7:15). As frustrating as it can feel, it's an intricate part of the journey. It's when we fail that we have the privilege of bowing before the Lord to confess, reconsider and regroup. Remember the words of James 1:3-4? *Consider it all joy when you encounter various trials, for the testing of your faith produces steadfastness. And let steadfastness have its full effect, that you may be perfect and complete, lacking in nothing.* I was ready to put my pride/anger/self-protection behind me, but it was too deeply ingrained to simply will it away. Clearly it was a trial, testing my faith, building steadfastness.

Are you ready to put your (un)health issues behind you, once and for all? Then celebrate the challenges. Don't forget, when you are weak, then He is strong. His power is perfected in your weakness. Plan to return to this section regularly.

Where/when did you recently "do that which you didn't want to do" in either the spiritual or physical realm? Which scriptures were you remiss in remembering? *Now* what promises will you claim? Write them out here:

_____

_____

_____

_____

Step back a moment and ask yourself, even though you are frustrated that you fumbled, has anything really changed? *All have sinned and fall short of the glory of God* (Romans 3:23). All you have to do is look around town to see lotsa folks are floundering. But as children of God, we have the Spirit-infused strength to get up, dust ourselves off and step back on track. Because it's easy to become discouraged by the difficulty of the journey, let's bear in mind a few Biblical truths.

Life is difficult.

Sorry saints, no one said this was going to be easy. In fact, as M. Scott Peck so memorably stated in his best-selling book, *The Road Less Traveled*, "Life is difficult." [Simon & Schuster, 1979] But don't trust Dr. Peck. Look at the Word of Truth:

For the gate is narrow and the way is hard that leads to life, and those who find it are few (Matthew 7:14).

In the world you will have tribulation. But take heart, I have overcome the world (John 16:33).

What physical disciplines do you find difficult, and why?

_____

_____

_____

_____

Listen into Miss Grace as she reminisces about God's unrelenting care, even during difficult times. https://www.livewellbygrace.com/speaking-blog/2019/10/7/beatitude

A Battle Rages

We all know – sort of – intellectually, at least – that Satan is out to get us. To knock us down. To render us ineffective for the Lord. But do you really believe that? If one of the reasons you want to better care for your temple is to increase your energy and enthusiasm for serving your Father, do you think the devil is going to sit back without a fight? Read the verses below to refresh your memory.

The thief comes only to steal and kill and destroy (John 10:10).

Be sober minded. Be watchful. Your adversary the devil prowls around like a roaring lion, seeking someone to devour. Resist him, firm in your faith, knowing that the same kinds of suffering are being experienced by your brotherhood throughout the world (1 Peter 5:8-9).

Cite several situations where you can imagine Satan is/was trying to sabotage you.

_____

_____

_____

. . . take up the whole armor of God, that you may be able to withstand in the evil day, and having done all, to stand firm.[14]*Stand therefore, having fastened on the belt of truth, and having put on the breastplate of righteousness,*[15]*and, as shoes for your feet, having put on the readiness given by the gospel of peace.*[16]*In all circumstances take up the shield of faith, with which you can extinguish all the flaming darts of the evil one;* (Ephesians 6:13-16).

When you're dodging Satan's darts, are you standing on Truth, or your feelings? Does your self-talk reflect what God says, or are you still listening to old, tired, untruthful tapes? Time to write:

_____

_____

_____

_____

_____

But the Lord is faithful. He will establish you and guard you against the evil one (2 Thessalonians 3:3).

Satan's arrows are whizzing past, and a couple nipped you. He's a formidable foe, that dog. But you've got a pinch hitter on your team. Not familiar with that term? Let's ask Wikipedia:

"In baseball, a pinch hitter is a substitute batter. Batters can be substituted at any time while the ball is dead (not in active play); the manager may use any player who has not yet entered the game as a substitute. Unlike basketball, American football, or ice hockey, baseball does not have a "free substitution rule" and thus the replaced player in baseball is not allowed back into that game. The pinch hitter assumes the spot in the batting order of the player whom he replaces."

It's the bottom of the last inning of the World Series and the score is 9-9. There are two outs, one man on base, and a rookie is up to bat. What's a coach to do? Put in a pinch hitter.

It's 7 p.m. and you just got home from work. It's been an unusually busy day with crazy colleagues and kids, and you haven't eaten since lunch. You're S-T-A-R-V-I-N-G! What do you do?

Put in a pinch hitter.

Let God go to bat.

'Cus if you try to defeat Satan in your own strength, you'll lose the game. Admit it. You're a rookie. Note: In this and all other challenges in life, you are permanently out of the game. Remember what Paul said in Colossians 3:3? *You died, and your life now is hidden with Christ in God.* Let Him bring in the win.

Are you familiar with Jehoshaphat's story in 2 Chronicles? There are three armies headed toward him with ill-intent. He prays, *We do not know what to do, but our eyes are on you.* Now there is a prayer that should be a post-it on your fridge. How many times every day are you confused about what to do? Call out to your Savior, "Lord, I don't know what to do, but my eyes are on you."

How do you think God responded to Jeho?

    a. He didn't.
    b. Good luck, I'm busy right now.
    c. You deserve to be obliterated.
    d. Do not be afraid nor be dismayed. The battle is not yours, but Mine.

What was that statement A.W. Tozer made? "What comes to our minds when we think about God is the most important thing about us." [A.W. Tozer, *The Knowledge of the Holy*]

So back to Jehoshaphat. How do you think God responded to him after he called out to Him in fear and humility? Yep, *Do not be afraid and do not be dismayed at this great horde, for the battle is not yours, but God's* (2 Chronicles 20:15).

Next time you're dodging the Devil's darts, pray like Jehoshaphat: "Lord, I don't know what to do, but my eyes are on you."

One of my favorite songs is "Ain't No Devil in Hell" by Danniebelle Hall. Listen to it here: https://www.youtube.com/watch?v=Hn1qEm57O4U

We are idolaters.

Strap in for this section; it's a tough one. We're going to take a peek into our hearts and honestly, it's not a pretty sight. Oh, we can all recite Romans 3:23 that says *all have sinned and fall short of the glory of God*, and we sort of intellectually agree with Paul's self-assessment, *for I know nothing good dwells in me* (Romans 7:18), and . . . *what a sinner I am!* (1 Corinthians 15:1-4; 1 Timothy 1:12-17). But the honest truth is, many of us don't really believe it. Just like Job, for the most part we think we're pretty nice folks. We go to church most Sundays, drop some dough in the offering plate, don't cheat, lie (well, maybe little ones...), or steal.

Human yearnings are a slippery slope. We tiptoe from a request to a demand in the blink of an eye. And if that demand isn't met, there's trouble in River City. Can you relate? You're up watching a sappy movie on Friday night and your brain nags, "A treat would be nice, something salty . . . or sweet. Maybe some ice cream?" Before you know it, you have lost track of the unfolding romance because you're obsessed with Rocky Road. Next thing you know you're on the road.

My idol of pride may manifest differently than your idol. My self-importance has many faces; it's revealed in multiple ways. Boastfulness. Greed. Unkindness. My favorite is love of comfort. The world must revolve around my good pleasure. One of my many self-protection ploys progressed from feeling safe only in solitude, to *requiring* a peaceful environment. How dare you disrupt my serenity with your lousy leaf blower! Quiet was no longer a request for me; it became a demand.

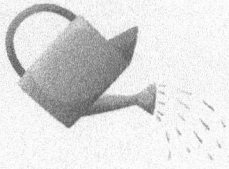

Stop Talking!

Paddling in the ocean in an outrigger canoe is magical. There's a reverent mantra to the synchronicity. Six paddles plunge into the water simultaneously, propelling the boat's nose through the surf. Each paddler twists at the torso and reaches long aside the seat ahead. Blades sweep just below the surface like an Olympic breast stroker, snap out at the hips, then quickly reach once more for the sea. Stroke . . . stroke . . . stroke . . . Like the tock of a sleepy metronome, the cadence is mesmerizing. The seagulls' squawk mystically meld into the mantra.

Unless someone's talking.

Paddling a six-man outrigger is certainly a social sport. All twelve hands are mandatory to move the monster from the boathouse to the beach. Because boys will be boys, conversation is always rife with jokes, jabs and jabber. Once on the water, even in the first minutes of warm-up, tales and teasing abound. But everyone understands that once the workout begins, it's all about timing, intensity, and focus.

Rick had been paddling for more decades than I'd been alive. As the steersman, he sat in seat six, which required skill vs. strength. It was second nature to him; as natural as breathing, which made him prone to blather. Ongoing inane comments. Dumb jokes. Life observations and opinions, none of which were welcome during workout.

Most of the guys just ignored him. "Oh, that's Rick. He never shuts up. You just have to tune him out."

But not Queen Judith. My mind was burning with rebuke. "How dare he! Shut up!" I couldn't paddle. I couldn't focus. The rhythm and reverence were broken. Recreation plummeted to reviling.

"Rick. Shhhhh . . . ," I not so subtly suggested.

Like the boat wake, my appeal washed away beyond the stern.

"Do you remember the time . . ." Rick reminisced.

Stroke . . . stroke . . . stroke . . . "Ignore him, Judith," I coaxed myself. "Stay in your zone. You are out in the ocean on a gorgeous Southern California morning, for gosh sakes. Are you going to let this crazy ol' coot steal your joy?" I was desperately trying to hold every thought captive, though my blood pressure was boiling.

Stroke . . . stroke . . . stroke . . .

"Feel your magnificent heart muscle working. What a glorious gift to have a strong, healthy cardiovascular system. Feel your back – your lats. Paddle in the strength of His spirit." My heart settled some.

"I remember in the late 80's at the San Diego race . . ."

"Seriously! Shut up! Shut the f&% up Rick!" I didn't say it, but I was losing it. I was about to turn around and push him off the back. "Can't he have some courtesy? Can he keep his mouth shut for ten minutes? Why isn't Pete saying anything? Why do they allow him to ruin our workout?" I was incensed. Enraged. My hostility only intensified my stroke.

Stroke . . . Stroke! . . . STROKE!

For a few minutes he shut up. Had he fallen overboard? I could only wish. "Settle down, Judith. Watch for dolphin. Notice the tides. The wind-whipped ripples on the water."

Stroke . . . stroke . . . stroke . . .

Stroke . . . stroke . . . stroke . . .

In perfect sync with the second person ahead*, I twisted my torso and dove my paddle into the water, pulling with full strength, then snapped it up and dropped it again.

Stroke . . . stroke . . . stroke . . .

"Hey Pete, where are we going for breakfast?"

I snapped.

---

* Unlike a rowing crew where each person pulls two oars (while facing backwards!), an outrigger paddle has a single face, so teammates paddle on alternate sides. Every 12-15 strokes, the person in seat two calls out "Hup!", the rest reply "Ho!" on the stroke following, then in unison everyone switches sides.

I shoved my paddle under the seat, threw my sunglasses into the bail bucket, and jumped overboard. For several seconds, like a run-away prisoner, I stayed below, pushing myself forward. Savoring the silence – the tranquility – I finally surfaced, gasping for air.

Despite my heaving, I could hear the boys' shouting.

Down again I dove, absorbing the calm of the deep. Stroke . . . stroke . . . stroke . . .

Up again for a reviving breath, then escaping to the underworld's stillness. Stroke . . . stroke . . . stroke . . .

The boys' calling, like the boat's wake, slowly disappeared into the distance. I was free to float atop the surf; to feel the cool water; to ingest the sea breeze. Keeping one eye on the lifeguard stand on the beach, my movements slowed, my breaths deepened, my anger subsided. The chaos was behind me. It was quiet. I was safe.

My belligerent bail out has become part of our canoe club lore, but I must recognize the revolting truth: I was committed to the kingdom of Judi. Like a petulant child, I am enraged if I don't get my way. My idol is my comfort, demanding quiet. I was paddling in the flesh – literally and spiritually – not in the Spirit.

Looking back, how would those boys describe me? Do they see me as a pleasant, loving, child of God? Hardly. They'd likely say, "She was quick to anger."

One of the many works of the flesh Paul lists in Galatians 5 is idolatry. Lest we skip over it to focus on seemingly more urgent faults (strife, jealousy, fits of anger) let's explore the meaning. We're going to access the wisdom of two very well-respected Christian brothers, David Powlison, former Executive Director of Christian Counseling Education Foundation (www.ccef.org), and Paul Tripp (www.PaulTripp.com). Below are a few of their insights:

> "There is an undeniable root and fruit connection between our heart and our behavior. People and situations do not determine our behavior; they provide the occasion where our behavior reveals our hearts . . . An idol of the heart is anything that rules me other than God . . . If God isn't ruling my heart, someone or something else will . . . Sin is fundamentally idolatrous. I do wrong things because my heart desires something more than the Lord . . . Our behavior is ruled, not by worship and service of the Lord, but by a ravenous desire for something . . . It [idolatry] steals the worship that rightly belongs to God and gives it to someone or something else . . . It is a life shaped by satisfaction of cravings . . . What we worship determines our responses to all of our experiences . . . Until the idol is removed, it will distort and obscure everything else in the person's life." [*Instruments in the Redeemers Hands*, Paul David Tripp, pp. 64-68]

> "We become engrossed in monstrous trivialities of our own devising." [*Seeing With New Eyes*, David Powlison p.78]

Rick's banal chatter sent me overboard, literally. Or was my behavior ruled by a ravenous, idolatrous desire for quiet? Was my prideful demand for peace an idol? Again:

> "There is an undeniable root and fruit connection between our heart and our behavior. People and situations do not determine our behavior; they provide the occasion where our behavior reveals our hearts" . . . "We become engrossed in monstrous trivialities of our own devising."

> "We were created to worship. It's in our DNA. The problem occurs when things like comfort, control and escape begin to function as gods for us. Turning to these counterfeit gods over and over again can have a cumulative effect on our lives. Over time we can become slaves to our own desires. This is the idolatry of addiction. In order to break free from this enslavement we must reorient our identity and replace the selfish desires of the heart with a new affection." [John Leonard, Founder & CEO, The Redemption House; www.redemptionhouse.net]

Wow. "The problem occurs when things like comfort, control and escape begin to function as gods for us. Turning to these counterfeit gods over and over again can have a cumulative effect on our lives. Over time we can become slaves to our own desires."

Ironically, my demand for comfort – insistence on serenity – had enslaved me.

Paul Tripp states, "An idol of the heart is anything that rules me other than God." What ruler do you worship like I did King Comfort? Does food rule you? Surely physical sustenance can't be an idol, can it? I mean, come on. A gal's gotta eat. Take these surveys, then reflect.

https://oa.org/quiz/
https://www.doctoroz.com/quiz/quiz-are-you-food-addict

Enlightening? What light bulb(s) have begun to flicker? Which questions gave you a tummy tremor? I get it. It's uncomfortable to stand before your Father and admit we've worshipped a false god. Stand up a minute. Take some deep breaths and raise your arms toward your Father. Tell Him how you're feeling. Stretch, refresh your coffee, then sit back down and muddle through your thoughts. Capture reasons, excuses, denials, hopes and dreams.

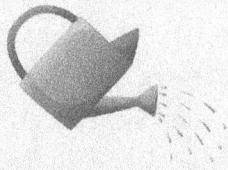

Quit Your Meanness

The title on the weathered spine screamed at me. *Quit Your Meanness* [Cranston & Stowe]. I pulled the vintage book from the shelf and sat down expectantly. Sam P. Jones was a 19th century preacher who didn't mince words. This treasure, published in 1886, was a compilation of several of his sermons. To my intrigue, the first was entitled *The City Wholly Given to Idolatry.* Sit down Judith, God has a word for you.

After dodging protests in Thessalonica, Paul found himself in Athens, and *his spirit was provoked within him as he saw that the city was full of idols.* He noted their alter "to the unknown god," then shared the good news about Jesus, the Christ. Pastor Jones compares first century Athens to 19th century America, which could be said two centuries along:

"I can take the daily papers of this city and read your local columns and see without getting at the Bible that it is wrong; that there is something radically wrong about it; there are too many debauched characters, too many suicides, too many murders, too many that are drifting daily to destruction and ruin. The fact is, a man doesn't need a Bible to see this world is all wrong; all you need to do is just to read your morning and afternoon papers, and then walk this street with your eyes open, and if you do that it will not be one week from today until you look on with horror that is indescribable.

Now let me ask each of you: Did you ever look at your heart until you saw it? I grant you that you have glanced at it a thousand times, but did you ever kneel down and pray for light, and look and look and look until you saw your heart? My Bible teaches me that: *The heart is deceitful above all things, and desperately wicked . . .* There is no such thing as a clean life outside of a clean heart."

I had to admit he was correct: my heart is deceitful and desperately wicked. Strangely, the confession gave me a sober sense of hope; the first step toward change is acknowledging the issue. Allegedly the late, great D.L. Moody prayed, "Lord God, show me my heart. Let me see it as it is."

Later in his sermon, Pastor Sam's words crumbled me again: "In the life of Jesus Christ, not a single harsh word ever escaped his lips toward a sinner. When Jesus would talk with a sinner, he would fetch up the parable of the lost sheep, where the man left the ninety and nine safe in the fold and followed the poor, wandering sheep, and when he found it he didn't take a club and beat it back home, but picked up the poor, tired, hungry sheep and laid it on his shoulder and brought it back to the fold."

That rattled me. It didn't sound like the Drill Sergeant Dad. He wouldn't beat me for my belligerence. He yearned to gently carry me back to the green pastures.

Lest we tumble down an emotional cliff, it is imperative we remember who we are in Christ. I loved and relied on Jesus, but hadn't been willing to deal with my judgment and anger. Maybe the surveys above prod you to deal with a blind spot, an idol of your own. I get snitty when my neighbor is being noisy; you get irritable when you can't eat what you crave. I rebel against authority and you against exercise, like a kid against green beans. Welcome to the world of being human. We are perhaps all prone to addiction – wanting something, like comfort, so compulsively we'll break God's commands to get it. But God's Word is clear. He wants us to want Him more than anything else.

Prone to Wander

"Prone to wander, Lord I feel it, prone to leave the God I love. Take my heart, Oh, take and seal it, with Thy Spirit from above." [*Come Thou Fount*, Robert Robinson, 1758]

Though clearly Tricia gave sage advice in 2010, I found myself back under her tutelage in 2020. I began writing *Sprinkled Clean* in the summer of 2018, all the while besieged by my besetting sin. The combination of an Internet installation fiasco to be revealed later, coupled with an unimaginably incompetent mortgage company and on-going car issues put me into a frenzy. I knew I needed a counseling refresher course. This time around, it quickly became clear my demons aren't unique. I can't shut down my anger with the snap of a finger any more than fitness strugglers can change their habits by mere resolve. So, when Tricia suggested I might want to consider a complete overhaul of this book, integrating my story, I thought I was going to wretch. Honestly, I was done. I had written, revised, and reorganized three times. Isn't that the tried-and-true formula for a charm? I was ready to *do* something – teach a class, create a curriculum, move along little doggies. Enough already with the revision. Let's wrap this up.

So not surprising, the subsequent three weeks were rife with distractions. As John Calvin so poignantly states, " . . . led away by any foolish hope or by any allurements, as many are hurried hither and thither by their own desires." [*Genesis*, Calvin, p. 109] Yep, I was hither and thithering all over the place.

Then it rained.

There are rainy days when you tuck in with a soft blanket and cup o' tea and read until you're cross-eyed, or settle contentedly into a Downton Abbey marathon. Then there are dark and gloomy days when God nails you. This drizzly Saturday, I got nailed.

Good and Angry*, by the beloved David Powlison, was Session 1. Noted below are a handful of Paternal shoulder shakes:

> "I want my way. When I don't get it, I make a stink . . . I'll punish anyone who crosses my will." (p. 17)

---

* *Good and Angry*, New Growth Press (September 12, 2016)

"You were ruled by your agenda, your expectations, your convenience, your pleasure, and your fears . . . when somebody or something got in your way, you lost it." (p. 20)

" . . . we can also get angry at the smallest thing that happens to go against what we want." (p. 40)

" . . . anger always makes a value judgment." (p. 41)

"Your desires become divine law . . . You have violated my will, and you deserve punishment." (p. 58)

If the shoe fits. Like Cinderella's slipper, Powlison's words were custom tailored for me.

The Second Act was authored by Anne Graham Lotz. *The Magnificent Obsession** uses Abraham's story to fine tune the readers' own. Passages that made my tummy hurt were:

"Abraham was not clear and decisive about fully following God's call." (p. 29)

"Abraham tried to do things God's way – and also his way. . . . he tried to force what he wanted and what God wanted in a synchronized plan. And it didn't work. Compromising with God never does." (p. 30)

"He was present in their lives whether or not they could see Him." (p. 38)

" . . . charging ahead without waiting for God's guidance." (p. 39)

" . . . very apprehensive about beginning again . . ." (p. 39)

"Instead of humbly submitting to His leadership, have you settled for achieving your own goals and dreams" (It's time to do something!) "Instead of investing your time in developing your personal relationship with God . . ." (p. 44)

"Abraham lost his peace, which is one of the hallmarks of someone who is wandering outside of God's will. A child of God who is outside of God's will becomes very insecure and has no confidence of God's presence or protection or provision." (p. 41) Translated, she's wandered from the green pastures, again . . .

OK, I get it. I'm not done with *Sprinkled Clean.*

And what's clear is my story, like yours, reveals multiple symptoms of the same sin. My impatience to cut short the work of the book is the same impatience that demands my way, lest I get angry. You disrupt my peace I get mad at you, because my highest

---

* *The Magnificent Obsession*, Zondervan; Reprint edition (August 28, 2010)

priority – my idol – is my comfort. Rewriting my/His book, again, was uncomfortable, not to mention the public processing of my insolence. I'd rather be distracted by building a Facebook following. The solution to both is the same: surrendering my heart to my Good Shepherd, trusting that all things work together for good, believing that He is doing a good work in me, and that His path, twists and turns included, is perfect.

Can you relate? You've become frustrated because you still haven't hit your ideal weight, so you're tempted to give up. Look at those thoughts and feelings here.

_____

_____

_____

Paul Tripp refers to those things that attract us – entrap us – consume us – as functional gods. They are the things that in the passion of the moment we want more than anything else, including God's call to self-care and self-control. They explain that ultimately our behavior is directed from our heart, not our mind or will. Only when the heart is transformed through the Spirit can we corral our compulsive behavior. Powlison says, "Your biggest problem is proud self-will." (p. 86) Tripp reinforces: "My choices and actions always reveal the desires that rule my heart." (p. 71)

Whether we are guilty of anger, impatience, selfishness, gluttony . . . doesn't it always come down to we want what we want and we're unhappy when we don't get it? " . . . we think of our lives as our own, and we are more committed to the purposes of our own kingdom than we are to God's." [*Instruments in the Redeemer's Hands*; Tripp; p. 106]

"Lasting change always takes place through the pathway of the heart. Fruit change is the result of root changes. Similarly, in Matthew 23, Christ says, *Clean the inside of the cup and dish and the outside will become clean.* Any agenda for change must focus on the thoughts and desires of the heart." [*Instruments*, p. 65]

Jeff Durbin, a reformed drug addict turned pastor of Apologia Church in Tempe, AZ says, "We don't have a drug, alcohol, sex, (food,) or gambling problem, we have a worship problem . . . The problem at bottom is rebellion."

Even John Calvin, a father to many faithful, allegedly said: "The human heart is an idol factory . . . Every one of us from our mother's womb is an expert in inventing idols."

So, there you have it. Our hearts *are* idolatrous. To be truly healed, we must acknowledge the only path to physical victory is heart surgery through surrender and sanctification.

This is tough stuff, gang. But don't be too hard on yourself. Everyone wants something more than they want God's will. Success. Notoriety. Quiet. Control. ("Lord, I'll follow as long as I get my way.") And remember, it's not that God doesn't want those things for us, but he wants our faith and satisfaction to be first in Him. Overcoming strongholds, whatever they are, always circles back to surrender. Aligning our wants and our will with God's commands. Paul Tripp says, "God changes us not just by teaching us to do different things, but by recapturing our hearts to serve Him alone." [*Instruments*, p. 71]

Ah ha! And therein lies the lie of diets. **Diets are about eating different foods; permanent, transformative change is about feasting regularly on the Bread of Life**.

Keeping our eyes on Jesus when we'd prefer to dive into an unhelpful comfort food isn't easy. As Dr. Tripp reinforces: "Every day creation battles with the Creator for the control of our hearts . . . .Whatever rules our hearts will control our behavior . . . horizontal desires (for people, possessions, recognition, control, acceptance, attention, vengeance, etc.) compete with the Lord for the rule of our hearts." [*Instruments*, p. 79]

Horizontal desires . . . food . . . sugar . . . comfort . . . compete with the Lord for the rule of our hearts.

Your dander and fists may be rising at this point. It seems so extreme! Food, an idol? Come on . . . But let's go back to either of the two previous surveys.

Do you think of food often . . . and get cranky when you are fasting from your favs? Describe.

_____

_____

Do you regularly schedule activities around food? Name a few.

_____

_____

Has it impacted your relationships? Your health? Explain how.

_____

_____

Are you constantly rebelling against exercise? Write your internal banter below. Now, in a sane moment, what do you think of that mental battle?

_____

_____

Now compare that to the amount of time and energy you spend in prayer and reading scripture. This is NOT about shaming, but what thoughts come up when you compare the two expenditures of time? What would you like to do to better balance the scale?

_____

_____

Go to a quiet place and pray, asking God to reveal idols in your heart. Grab a box of Kleenex and record your conversation here.

_____

_____

_____

_____

_____

_____

Call It Out

Powlison and Tripp are quite clear that it is idolatry that derails us, leaving us impotent, frustrated, dejected, . . . But what's your "it"? What is it you want in the moment of temptation more than you want God's best? To what false god(s) do you bow? Fear, anger, depression, control, gluttony, lust of the flesh . . . Our primary focus here is food and fitness, but oftentimes that's merely a symptom of the real, deep, heartfelt yearning. Is it love? Companionship? Acknowledgement? Remember, when we want them more than we want God's will, these hungers of the heart become "functional gods." It's your internal control panel that directs your thoughts, actions, and emotions. Below the boys set the stage for inner excavation.

> "As a Christian you profess that God controls all things, and works everything to his glory and your ultimate well-being. You profess that God is your rock and refuge, a very present help in whatever troubles you face. You profess to worship him, trust him, love him, obey him. But in that moment – or hour, day, season – of anxiety, you live as if you needed to control all things. You live as if something – money, someone's approval, a "successful" sermon, your grade on an exam, good health, avoiding conflict, getting your way – matters

more than trusting and loving God. You live as if some temporary good feeling could provide you refuge, as if your actions could make the world right. Your functional god competes with your professed God. Unbelievers are wholly owned by ungodly motives – their functional gods. Yet true believers are often severely compromised, distracted, and divided by our functional gods as well. Thankfully, grace reorients us, purifies us, and turns us back to our Lord. Grace makes our professed God and functional God one and the same." [*Seeing With New Eyes,* David Powlison, pp. 130-131]

Why do all this digging? For the " . . . reorientation of motives through the grace of the Gospel." (Ibid)

If you are truly committed to uncovering your motivations, please get *Seeing With New Eyes*, even if you only read the X-Ray Questions in Chapter 7. Powlison presents a series of probing questions that drill deep into the bedrock of your soul. One example, "What do you want, desire, crave, lust, and wish for? What desires do you serve and obey?" (He could compete with Joyce Meyer for the Call-It-Like-You-See-It Award.)

Go to a quiet place to complete this next exercise. You may want to go out under the oak tree or to your favorite hide-away. Regardless of your response, it's all OK. You are on the road to living life abundantly.

Consider the last three times you chose unhealthy foods or avoided exercise. Describe the circumstances and your *real* reason for compromising.

1. _____
_____
_____

2. _____
_____
_____

3. _____
_____
_____

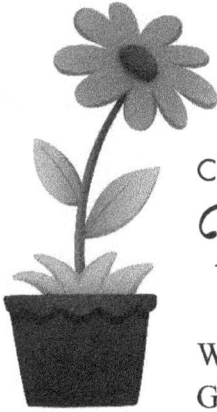

CHAPTER 4
Embrace Grace

We now know we're idolaters. Nice. What do we do with that? Grab God's grace. Hebrews 4:16 says, *Let us then with confidence draw near to the throne of grace, that we may receive mercy and find grace to help in time of need.* We sing, "Your grace is enough," but do we believe it? Are we fully convinced His Spirit, by His grace, can transform our earthly passions into the fruit of self-discipline? Consider again the words of David Powlison:

> "No one can truly change who does not know and rely on gifts from the hand of the Lord. Since Christ is both Giver and Gift, attempts to change without grace are barren of the very purpose, power, and Person that change is about. Self-manufactured changes do not dislodge almighty me from the center of my tiny self-manufactured universe. Still in the futility of my mind and the hardness of my heart, I only act a bit different. Successful living without grace describes mere self-reformation; get your act together, save your marriage, get off your duff and get a job. Failure in living describes failed self-efforts: when you can't get a grip, you despair. Christ-less, grace-less attempts to change conclude either with the praise of your own glory or with your shame." [*Seeing With New Eyes,* David Powlison, p. 48]

Wow. There it is. It's not about my efforts or intentions. My willpower will always fail at some point. It always goes back to God and His grace. It is too high. I cannot attain it.

Tripp reinforces, "It is important to remember the new character qualities and behavior patterns that are in your life because of Jesus. You already have a new heart. You have been radically changed by his grace and are being progressively restored day by day. That is the focus of God's work in your life right now.

The only way to properly celebrate these realities is to humbly ask, 'God, where are you calling me to further change? What qualities that you promise to your children are still not active in my heart? What do you want me to see about you?'" [*How People Change,* Paul Tripp, p. 117]

STOP! and reflect: Answer Pastor Paul's questions above, both generally and relative to your health choices.

_____

_____

_____

For the grace of God has appeared, bringing salvation for all people, training us to renounce ungodliness and worldly passions, and to live self-controlled, upright, and godly lives in the present age (Titus 2:11-12).

What does this verse mean to you, specifically relative to your fitness efforts?

_____

_____

_____

It's important here to remember the difference between justification and sanctification, both achieved *only* by God's grace. Justification is our salvation into eternal life by accepting Jesus Christ as our Lord and Savior. Sanctification is the subsequent lifelong process of growing in Christ-likeness. Justification happens once; sanctification is a forever process this side of heaven. Though a newborn babe is fully human, he must grow physically and spiritually to reach his full potential. This comparison provides insight into Jesus' statement to Nicodemus, *Truly, truly, I say to you unless one is born again, he cannot see the kingdom of God (*John 3:3). For an insightful differentiation and explanation on justification vs. sanctification, listen to this sermon by David Platt at McLean Bible Church in Washington DC: https://radical.net/sermon/the-cross-and-christian-sanctification/

A notable verse speaking to the sanctification process is 2 Corinthians 3:18: *And we all, with unveiled face, beholding the glory of the Lord, are being transformed into the same image from one degree of glory to another. For this comes from the Lord who is the Spirit.*

What does this verse tell us? As we behold the glory of the Lord, we are slowly – *from one degree of glory to another* – transformed into His image, through His Spirit.

Once again, David Platt says it succinctly: "We become what we behold. Where we focus our minds comes out in our lives. The more we look to Christ, the more we'll look like Christ."

Take a moment to ponder those statements. How might you behold Him more, and how would that impact your fitness process?

_____

_____

_____

Let's go back to Powlison:

"The only way you can wrestle yourself down is by the promises of God. You need help the way a drowning man needs help from outside himself to rescue him . . . .We escape ourselves by being loved by Jesus Christ through the powerful presence of the Holy Spirit." [*Seeing with New Eyes,* David Powlison. pp. 81-82]

We keep circling around the concept of "We can't, but He can." It's a tough lesson. Where are you still trying and not trusting?

_____

_____

_____

1 John 5:14-15 reads: [14]*And this is the confidence that we have toward him, that if we ask anything according to his will he hears us.* [15]*And if we know that he hears us in whatever we ask, we know that we have the requests that we have asked of him.*

If you believe God wants you to better tend your temple, do you think He's prepared to help? If so, is seeking His assistance your pathway to success and sanity? What are your next right steps?

_____

_____

_____

Seen by Grace

Let's take a moment to consider how God sees His children. *After you believed in Him as LORD and were sealed in the Holy Spirit* (Eph 1:13), He sees you with new eyes. Like a Hollywood diet, let's peek at the before and after photo.

A Father's Eyes: Pre-Christ

It is a bit embarrassing to muse on the mess we were before Christ grabbed us. We prefer to ponder reconciliation, forgiveness and freedom. At the risk of offending anyone, the following reinforce our previously pathetic state. Read through them and jot down words and phrases that jolt you.

Spiritually dead – Ephesians 2:1-3

_____

Everyone is corrupt – Psalm 14:2-3

_____

Enemies of God – Ephesians 2:3; Romans 5:10

_____

Idol worshipper – Colossians 3:7

_____

A Father's Eyes: In Christ

But God . . . *so loved the world that He gave his only son that whosoever believeth on Him shall not perish but have everlasting life* (John 3:16).

"Amazing Grace, how sweet the sound, that saved a wretch like me." [*Amazing Grace*, John Newton, 1772]

When I was in one of my rebellious phases, I refused to say "wretch" when singing Amazing Grace in church. "I'm not a wretch! How demeaning!" With blood pressure boiling, I sang, "who saved a child like me." Like many unrepentant Christians, I saw myself as a pretty good egg, far from a corrupt, idol-worshipping, enemy of God. But God doesn't grade on the curve. We church-going, Bible-reading, tithe-paying, Jesus-followers are clearly described in the previous passages. *All* have sinned. No one makes the grade. Everyone is doomed to hell unless they surrender their life to Jesus. AND God sees my snitty, self-serving spirit as every bit as loathsome as "those people's" problems. When was the last time you humbly bowed before your Father, thanking Him for saving you?

Not only are we assured we'll spend eternity with Him, consider how this loving, redeeming, full-of-grace God thinks about us now. Read Ephesians 1:3-14 and list all the blessings and benefits you find:

_____

_____

_____

After earlier acknowledging our tendency toward self-satisfying idols, it is humbling to list these blessings and benefits, isn't it? It's difficult to fathom that God now sees us through His lens of grace. In His eyes we are a new creation, born again, free from the bondage of the flesh. Our sole purpose on earth is to reflect Christ, for God's glory. From His perspective, we are already *being transformed into the same image from one degree of glory to another.*

"Begin with the end in mind," said Ken Blanchard in his best-selling book, *The One Minute Manager*. Though turns out, that wasn't a novel concept. Jesus said in John 20:29, *blessed are those who believe before they see.* Let's muse a minute at how God sees His beloved children.

A New Creation

2 Corinthians 5:17 says, *Therefore, if anyone is in Christ, he is a new creation. The old has passed away; behold, the new has come.* As we fumble in our foibles, it's tough to see ourselves as a "new creation." Sinful habits don't give up the ghost easily. As we stumble toward sanctification, we must keep our eye on the prize; remain steadfastly focused on who we are in Christ, based not on our feelings but on God's calling.

Pastor John MacArthur (www.gty.org) offers an excellent analogy for understanding our standing as a new creation, using the comparison of position and practice. Consider the star quarterback of your favorite football team. His definitive position is the team's key player. Your definitive position, confirmed by the holy scriptures, is a new creation. You are holy, partaking in the Divine nature.

Mr. Quarterback practices his position. If he consistently throws incomplete passes, gets sacked, and/or calls unwise plays, he becomes ineffective and may be benched, or worse. You and I must practice our position too. *Be ye holy as I AM holy.* "Practice is where the growth is, becoming who you are," says MacArthur. Remember, salvation is immediate; renewal is on-going. Like that baby who has all the necessary parts to be fully human, he still needs to grow to meet his full potential. Hebrews 5:14 says, *But solid food is for the mature, for those who have their powers of discernment trained by constant practice to distinguish good from evil.* Practice your position! (We'll talk more in Chapter 8 about how to practice.)

What bubbles up inside you when you tell yourself you are a new creation in Christ?

_____

_____

_____

Chosen, Adopted Children

Ephesians 1:5-6 says *He predestined us for adoption to himself as sons through Jesus Christ.* Adoption was a big deal in ancient times, because an adopted child had all the privileges of a biological child, irrevocable forever. Even today, during the court process, adoptive parents must testify they understand they are making a lifelong commitment, and intend to provide the child a safe, loving home. Real parents never make that pledge! Understanding my adoption by Christ was one of the primary principals that helped me envision transformation. I wasn't a child of an abusive father; I was the child of the Almighty God who *chose* me. Picked me for His team. Pulled me out of the pit and brought me into His house. Though I had questioned His goodness, clearly He had provided exceeding abundantly greater than I could ever think or imagine. By His mercy, I wasn't destined to struggle forever financially; I was simply in a valley along my God-ordained path toward transformation.

Rex Cole from The Village Church in Dallas, TX, tells the story of an American couple who did an international adoption from an orphanage. The child had been living in deplorable conditions, including sleeping on the floor. When the boy first arrived, the father would go into his room at night to tuck him in and would find him lying in the corner, on the floor. He had to explain to the young boy that he had been adopted into their family – that their home was his new home – and that he no longer, and never would again, have to sleep on the floor.

Even though you have been adopted into a safe, comfortable home with a soft, warm bed, are there areas in your life where you're still sleeping on the floor? Describe.

_____

_____

_____

Though the Word refers to God as Father, do you trust Him as yours? If your earthly father was less than loving, is it tough for you to imagine your heavenly Father is trustworthy and safe? Be honest here.

_____

_____

_____

_____

Let's face it. A choice is . . . well . . . a choice. God wasn't forced to pick us. He could have left us doomed to destruction. But like a loving Father, He sent His Son to lift us out of the pit.

For all who are led by the Spirit of God are sons of God. For you did not receive the spirit of slavery to fall back into fear, but you have received the Spirit of adoption as sons, by whom we cry, Abba! Father! The Spirit himself bears witness with our spirit that we are children of god, and if children, then heirs – heirs of God and fellow heirs with Christ (Romans 8:14-16).

Do you believe this? Why? Why not? What part?

_____

_____

How do you feel about the idea of being chosen? Explain how it impacts who you are and how you see the world.

_____

_____

United with Christ

But he who is joined to the Lord becomes one spirit with him (1 Corinthians 6:17).

One spirit with Jesus. Ponder that a minute. It's tough to comprehend when we still get sidetracked by low blood sugar, road rage and P.M.S. I always find personalizing scripture helpful, and there it is in black and white. *She who is joined to the Lord becomes one spirit with Him.* Chew on that truth in the first person throughout your day today. "I am one spirit with Jesus."

Life offers a handful of examples of living united with another. Marriage is the most obvious. Anyone with a twin sibling understands connectedness. Sports teams, some working relationships, and hopefully church congregations experience the benefits of being allied. If you are united with Christ, one spirit with Him as 1 Corinthians 6:17 says, how does it impact your daily journey?

_____

_____

Redeemed, Forgiven and FREE!

I will walk at liberty: for I seek Thy precepts (Psalm 119:45, KJV).

As I've admitted, freedom is a BIG deal to me. I want my way, on my terms. But the possibility that I was actually in bondage to my anger began to bother me. If I'm not getting what I want I'll scream at you, but afterwards I feel like a heel. I wanted to be free indeed, and all roads to recovery led back to Calvary.

. . . He has blessed us in the Beloved. In him we have redemption through his blood, the forgiveness of our trespasses, according to the riches of his grace, which he lavished upon us in all wisdom and insight, making known to us the mystery of his will . . . (Ephesians 1:6-7).

[18]All this is from God, who through Christ reconciled us to himself and gave us the ministry of reconciliation; [19]that is, in Christ God was reconciling the world to himself, not counting their trespasses against them, and entrusting to us the message of reconciliation (2 Corinthians 5:18-19).

Redeem means to buy back; to free from captivity by payment of ransom. Jesus died for me, yet all I want is my way. Tricia's words haunted me. "If He did nothing else, He has done more then you deserve." I had to search my soul and ask, what did my redemption really mean to me?

I never really understood the first beatitude. *Blessed are the poor in spirit, for theirs is the kingdom of heaven* (Matthew 5:3). Does that mean we're supposed to go through life downtrodden and depressed? Heaven forbid. But it does refer to this idea of contrite gratitude for our salvation. Powlison defines poor in spirit as "conscious awareness of dire and pressing need for help that God most freely and generously gives." [*God's Grace and Your Sufferings*, Christian Counseling and Educational Foundation, ccef.org]

This visual of humble acknowledgement of our profound need not only relates to our salvation, but to conquering our daily sins.

What does your redemption mean to you? How does it impact your daily decisions, including your food and fitness choices?

_____

_____

_____

Read Colossians 1:21-23. Synonyms to reconcile are reunite, bring together, make peace. Did you have a "former life" story from which you are grateful to be free and forgiven? Write about it here.

_____

_____

Though God is at peace with your days of alienation, are you? Have you accepted his full forgiveness? Share any lingering guilt pangs.

_____

_____

God's Workmanship

Before reading the following verses, pull out your Bible and slowly read through Psalm 139. What verses stand out to you and why?

_____

_____

[10] *For we are his workmanship, created in Christ Jesus for good works, which God prepared beforehand, that we should walk in them (Ephesians 2:10).*

[26] *Then God said, "Let us make man in our image, after our likeness. And let them have dominion over the fish of the sea and over the birds of the heavens and over the livestock and over all the earth and over every creeping thing that creeps on the earth." [27] So God created man in his own image, in the image of God he created him; male and female he created them (Genesis 1:26-27).*

After turning on the lights, separating land and sea, making trees, cattle and bees, God made man in His image. Imagine yourself a reflection of God. How does this divine design impact your perception of your body?

_____

_____

_____

Body image can be a tough conversation. "I hate how I look," say many. Sometimes it's her nose, or thighs, or bum – and today, seems kids are even questioning their sex. But how can that be when God was the general contractor for your construction project? Your frame was not secret from God Almighty, when you were being made – intricately woven.

There's a pithy statement out there, God doesn't make junk. Candidly, it's true.

Now we all know and must admit, our job is to care for that body, and it wants real, God-grown food and regular movement. Choices can change our original condition. But the good news is, just like God is forgiving, so are our bodies. If you've not followed the Manufacturers Instructions, it's not too late to start.

Righteous and Holy

Re-read Colossians 1:21-23. Through Jesus' death, we are presented holy and blameless and above reproach before God. Sit with that a minute. What feelings bubble up?

_____

_____

_____

I don't know about you but given all I've shared, it's tough for me to see myself as righteous and holy. If you asked my friends, "Name three adjectives that describe Judi," neither righteous nor holy would likely make the top 100. Do you feel the same? "Righteous? Holy? Me? Who are you kidding?" Yep, it's a hard one to swallow. Fortunately, God sees you and me through the sacrifice of Jesus. Remember, _He chose us in him before the foundation of the world, that we should be holy and blameless before him_ (Eph. 1:4). Holy doesn't mean we're perfectly pure, but that we're "set apart, dedicated." We have been cleansed through Christ. We are new creations, not because of anything we've done, but because of what *Jesus* did. *"He is the propitiation for our sins,"* says I John 2:2. We have been cleansed by the blood of the lamb. Embrace His grace.

When I placed my anger alongside the idea of being a new creation, there was definitely a disconnect. Like an old shoe with a loose heel flapping with every step, (But they're still good lawn mowing shoes!) it was time for it to go.

How does it feel to know God sees you as righteous and holy? How can you step into it?

_____

_____

_____

How can you embrace that truth and let it impact your food and fitness choices and resolve?

_____

_____

_____

Known

After meditating earlier on God's glory, it's hard to fathom that God intimately knows us, isn't it? He knows the number of hairs on our head (Matt 10:30-31), and when we sit down and get up (Psalm 139:2). Reflect on Psalm 139:2-4, marveling that you are known by the One who holds all those galaxies in His hand: *You discern my thoughts from afar. You search out my path and my lying down and are acquainted with all my ways. Even before a word* (thought) *is on my tongue, behold, O Lord, you know it altogether.*

One more time let's ponder the passage, phrase by phrase. When you look back at your struggle to change your food habits and step up your exercise, consider each of the phrases below, noting how it relates to your physical journey:

You discern my thoughts from afar

_____

You search out my path

_____

You are acquainted with all my ways

_____

You know all I think, say, and do (and don't do . . .)

_____

If God is indeed intimately acquainted with all your ways, do you see that as good news, or not so much?

_____

_____

What does it mean to you to be "known" by the Father? What do you want Him to know – notice – and to what would you like Him to turn a blind eye? Honestly, I wasn't thrilled he knew by name all the customer service reps I'd ripped . . .

_____

_____

I am the good shepherd. I know my own and my own know me, just as the Father knows me and I know the Father; and I lay down my life for the sheep (John 10:14-15).

Do you see Him as a Good Shepherd, trustworthy of your whole heart, including the part that's angry, scared, lonely, confused? Talk to Him here.

_____

_____

Miss Grace relishes her good buddy Mildred, comparing her faithful friendship with His. https://www.livewellbygrace.com/speaking-blog/2019/8/5/remembered

Temple of the Holy Spirit

The Word is clear that when you accepted Christ as your Lord and Savior, the Spirit entered you. Read below:

[13]*In him you also, when you heard the word of truth, the gospel of your salvation, and believed in him, were sealed with the promised Holy Spirit,* [14]*who is the guarantee of our inheritance until we acquire possession of it, to the praise of his glory* (Ephesians 1:13-14).

²¹And it is God who establishes us with you in Christ, and has anointed us, ²²and who has also put his seal on us and given us his Spirit in our hearts as a guarantee (2 Corinthians 1:21-22).

The Holy Spirit is the least discussed and most misunderstood of the divine Trinity. We revere God Almighty, we cling to Christ as Savior, but we're not exactly sure what to do with the Holy Spirit. We vaguely acknowledge He's "inside us," that He helps guide and chide us, but beyond that most don't give Him much thought. The scriptures are clear the Spirit should play more than a bit part in our spiritual drama. Read the following passages and note His work:

John 14:15-27 _____

John 16:5-15 _____

Romans 8:1-27 (Oh, go ahead. Read the entire chapter.)

What did you learn about the third Providential Pillar? (Answers below – don't peek!)

_____

_____

He is your Helper. (John 14:16-17, John 16:7)

Your Comforter. (John 14:27)

He will guide you. (John 16:13)

He brings to your remembrance things you've learned about God. (John 14:26)

He helps you pray and intercedes for you. (Romans 8:26-27)

He helps you to stop sinning. (Romans 8:1-6) This is gonna come in handy . . .

If you believe the Holy Spirit lives in you, how does that impact your thoughts, words, and actions?

_____

_____

Appendix 2 offers several verses I call "Royalty Reminders". In a world that tells us we're not _____ enough, (Fill in your own falsehood: smart, spiritual, successful . . .) we must constantly remind ourselves who we are in Christ.

We must battle Satan's lies through memorization of truth. Print the list and keep it handy. Read your favorites again and again, and watch the Spirit transform you.

All would be wise to heed the warning God gave the Israelites in Deuteronomy 8:11-14:

Take care lest you forget the Lord your God by not keeping his commandments and his rules and his statutes, which I command you today, *[12]lest, when you have eaten and are full and have built good houses and live in them,* *[13]and when your herds and flocks multiply and your silver and gold is multiplied and all that you have is multiplied,* *[14]then your heart be lifted up, and you forget the Lord your God, who brought you out of the land of Egypt, out of the house of slavery,*

Let us *never* forget. God saved us. He pulled us from the miry bog. We did nothing – NO thing – to deserve it and could never earn it. By grace alone, through faith alone, in Christ alone, we have been saved.

Embrace your inheritance in Christ, beloved, . . . *that you may know what is the hope to which He has called you, what are the riches of His glorious inheritance in the saints . . .* (Ephesians 1:18).

Yes, but . . .

All the above likely got a knowing, grateful, nod. But if you're like me, you're thinking, yes, but . . . Trust me, I understand.

Earning God's Love

Naaman had it goin' on. A Syrian army commander with a history of combat victory, he was in the king's inner circle and good graces, not to mention, loaded. A prime candidate for pride. . . . *but he was a leper* (2 Kings 5:1). Five life-altering words.

After his aforementioned battle win, Naaman kidnapped a young Israeli girl to be his wife's servant. When the girl heard about his leprosy, instead of holding revengeful gratification, she told her mistress of a prophet in Samaria who could cure his disease.

Let's stop there. A brutal dictator overtakes your country, does who-knows-what to your family, then kidnaps you into slavery. If he were your boss, would you try to help him? Just sayin', I wouldn't.

Instead of going to the prophet, though, Naaman loads up his buggy with silver, gold, and gifts, and heads to the Syrian king. He tells the king what the young girl said, then left with a royal introduction to the Israeli king. Naaman's strategy was obviously,... Why go to a lowly prophet when you can lobby a Ruler? Their strategy was obviously, "It's not what you know but who you know." Why go to a prophet when you can go right to the Ruler?

But the Israeli king was befuddled. *Am I God, to kill and to make alive, that this man sends word to me to cure a man of his leprosy?* (2 Kings 5:7).

News travels fast in a small town, so when the prophet Elisha, who the servant girl had recommended, heard someone had contacted the king for a cure, he messaged him, *Let him*

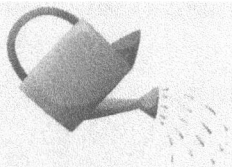

Earning God's Love

Though I had been sufficiently pummeled by David Powlison and Paul Tripp over my fruitless functional gods, I picked up Tim Keller's book, *Counterfeit Gods*. Chapter Four brought me to tears. He begins by quoting an article written about award-winning film director Sydney Pollack who said, "Every time I finish a picture, I feel like I've done what I'm supposed to do in the sense that I've earned my stay for another year or so." I was stunned. That was me. For thirty years I pushed and pushed and pushed, trying to earn my keep.

Then Keller muses on Naaman. "Naaman expected that Elisha would take the money and perform some magic ritual. Or, he thought, if Elisha did not take the money, he would at least demand that Naaman do 'some great thing' to *earn* his healing. Instead he was asked to simply go and dip himself seven times in the Jordan River. At this he went off in a rage. . . . Now he was being confronted with a God who in his dealings with human beings only operates on the basis of grace." [*Counterfeit Gods*, Penguin Books, p. 87]

The tears trickled. I wasn't trying to earn my salvation. I knew that Jesus died for sinners like me, and I had humbly accepted His sacrifice. But . . . *I was trying to earn His love*. Like Naaman, I was prepared to pay for the gracious gift. Pray and read His Word. Tithe. Write a book. I did those things because I truly loved my Lord, but still, grace was hard for me to grasp. He'd take note of my efforts, right? Would He still love me if I didn't do them? What if I spent my retirement years riding my bike and reading fanciful fiction? Would God still love me?

Seems I'm not alone in this misguided thinking. In his heart-softening book, *Transforming Grace*, Jerry Bridges writes: "Our expectation of God's blessing depends on how well we feel we are living the Christian life . . . we innately think so much performance by us earns so much blessing from God . . . .One of the best kept secrets among Christians today is this: *Jesus paid it all. I mean all. He not only purchased your forgiveness of sins and your ticket to heaven, He purchased every blessing and every answer to prayer you will ever receive.* [*Transforming Grace*, NavPress, pp. 16-18]

My head was spinning. Where's the balance between serving the Lord in love, and trying to earn His affection? Bridges acknowledges and addresses my confusion: "Then we turn to the Bible and read that we are to work out our salvation, to pursue holiness, and to be diligent to add to our faith such virtues as goodness, knowledge, self-control, and love. In fact, we find the Bible filled with exhortations to do good works and pursue the disciplines of spiritual growth. Again, because we are legalistic by nature, we assume our performance in these areas earns God's blessings in our lives."

Having been reared by a disciplinarian father, I was an accomplished, calculated, favor-earner. "9:00 means 8:55 . . ." Seven A's and one B on a report card wasn't good enough for Dad. Lord, how can I be good enough for You? If I . . . . will I be good enough? *Are you so foolish? Having begun by the Spirit, are you now being perfected by the flesh?* (Galatians 3:3). "If Elisha did not take the money, he would at least demand that Naaman do 'some great thing' to *earn* his healing. Instead he was asked to simply go and dip himself seven times in the Jordan River." But Lord, I can do more than that! Anyone can just jump in the suds. I could do great things for You . . . "He was being confronted with a God who in his dealings with human beings only operates on the basis of grace." *But if it is by grace, it is no longer on the basis of works; otherwise grace would no longer be grace* (Romans 11:6). "9:00 means 8:55 . . ." "What happened there?" Dad looking at the B in disdain. "We're going to look for your father."

His steadfast love endures forever.

Lord, forgive me for believing I need to earn your love – trying to be good enough. And for my pride in believing there is absolutely anything I could do or give that would be worthy. Like Naaman, if I earn it, I'm not beholden to anyone. My feet are still on solid ground. I'm in control. I'm safe . . . but not surrendered.

come now to me, that he may know that there is a prophet in Israel. Elisha knew an opportunity when he saw one.

Begrudgingly, Naaman and his entourage went to Elisha, but the prophet didn't even have the courtesy to come to the door. He simply sent a messenger saying, "Go wash in the Jordan seven times."

Naaman was offended and fuming. "Don't you know who I am?" He was prepared to write a big check, and the guy doesn't even show him the respect of greeting him. He turned on his heels in a huff.

Naaman's servants had surely seen this prideful side of him, but still they suggested, *My father, if the prophet had told you to do some great thing, would you not have done it? How much more, then, when he tells you, 'Wash and be cleansed'!* (NIV) Naaman conceded, and went to the river to wash. *His flesh was restored like the flesh of a little child, and he was clean.*

Though I had been sufficiently pummeled by David Powlison and Paul Tripp over my fruitless functional gods, I picked up Tim Keller's book, *Counterfeit Gods.* Chapter Four brought me to tears. He begins by quoting an article written about award-winning film director Sydney Pollack who said, "Every time I finish a picture, I feel like I've done what I'm supposed to do in the sense that I've earned my stay for another year or so." I was stunned. That was me. For thirty years I pushed and pushed and pushed, trying to earn my keep.

Then Keller muses on Naaman. "Naaman expected that Elisha would take the money and perform some magic ritual. Or, he thought, if Elisha did not take the money, he would at least demand that Naaman do 'some great thing' to *earn* his healing. Instead he was asked to simply go and dip himself seven times in the Jordan River. At this he went off in a rage. . . . Now he was being confronted with a God who in his dealings with human beings only operates on the basis of grace." [*Counterfeit Gods*, Penguin Books, p. 87]

The tears trickled. I wasn't trying to earn my salvation. I knew that Jesus died for sinners like me, and I had humbly accepted His sacrifice. But . . . *I was trying to earn His love.* Like Naaman, I was prepared to pay for the gracious gift. Pray and read His Word. Tithe. Write a book. I did those things because I truly loved my Lord, but still, grace was hard for me to grasp. He'd take note of my efforts, right? Would He still love me if I didn't do them? What if I spent my retirement years riding my bike and reading fanciful fiction? Would God still love me?

Seems I'm not alone in this misguided thinking. In his heart-softening book, *Transforming Grace,* Jerry Bridges writes: "Our expectation of God's blessing depends on how well we feel we are living the Christian life . . . we innately think so much performance by us earns so much blessing from God . . . .One of the best kept secrets among Christians today is this: *Jesus paid it all. I mean all. He not only purchased your forgiveness of sins and your ticket to heaven, He purchased every blessing and every answer to prayer you will ever receive.* [*Transforming Grace*, NavPress, pp. 16-18]

My head was spinning. Where's the balance between serving the Lord in love, and trying to earn His affection? Bridges acknowledges and addresses my confusion: "Then we turn to the Bible and read that we are to work out our salvation, to pursue holiness, and to be diligent to add to our faith such virtues as goodness, knowledge, self-control, and love. In fact, we find the Bible filled with exhortations to do good works and pursue the disciplines of spiritual growth. Again, because we are legalistic by nature, we assume our performance in these areas earns God's blessings in our lives."

Having been reared by a disciplinarian father, I was an accomplished, calculated, favor-earner. "9:00 means 8:55 . . ." Seven A's and one B on a report card wasn't good enough for Dad. Lord, how can I be good enough for You? If I . . . . will I be good enough? *Are you so foolish? Having begun by the Spirit, are you now being perfected by the flesh?* (Galatians 3:3). "If Elisha did not take the money, he would at least demand that Naaman do 'some great thing' to *earn* his healing. Instead he was asked to simply go and dip himself seven times in the Jordan River." But Lord, I can do more than that! Anyone can just jump in the suds. I could do great things for You . . . "He was being confronted with a God who in his dealings with human beings only operates on the basis of grace." *But if it is by grace, it is no longer on the basis of works; otherwise grace would no longer be grace* (Romans 11:6). "9:00 means 8:55 . . ." "What happened there?" Dad looking at the B in disdain. "We're going to look for your father."

His steadfast love endures forever.

Lord, forgive me for believing I need to earn your love – trying to be good enough. And for my pride in believing there is absolutely anything I could do or give that would be worthy. Like Naaman, if I earn it, I'm not beholden to anyone. My feet are still on solid ground. I'm in control. I'm safe . . . but not surrendered.

Have you ever found yourself trying to earn God's favor, forgetting it's freely given by grace? My brain was congested with this conundrum. In search of encouragement on another nagging issue, waiting on God, John Piper swept open the blackout curtains. In his sermon at Christ Redeemer Church in Woodbury, MN on May 5, 2013, Piper opened with Isaiah 64:1-4. Verse 4 reads, *From of old no one has heard or perceived by the ear, no eye has seen a God besides you, who acts for those who wait for him.* My unsettledness over waiting on something began to dissipate. But as he continued, God gave clarity on my foolish attempts to earn Gods love. Piper said, "God's greatness is not magnified by workers to work for Him, but His greatness is magnified by working for His people." He based this statement on Acts 17:25 which says *nor is He served by human hands, as though He needed anything, since He himself gives to all mankind life and breath and everything.* "You don't serve Him; He serves you." Piper

The tornado in my brain whipped up again. God almighty, set to serve me? That can't be right. Pastor John must misunderstand.

He continued with a terrific analogy. A warehouse in his neighborhood had a Help Wanted sign permanently affixed to the building. Periodically, though, a big red NO would be mounted, declaring their complete personnel roster. In typical exuberant Piper fashion, he shouts, "That's the gospel! God never hangs out a Help Wanted sign. He doesn't need our help! In fact, His sign would read 'Help Available'!"

Per usual, he presented additional scriptures to reinforce his point. *For the eyes of the LORD run to and fro throughout the whole earth, to give strong support to those whose heart is blameless toward Him* (2 Chronicles 16:9). The New International Version says *for those whose hearts are fully committed to Him.* God wants to help us – to give us His strong support. I was reminded of Isaiah 26:3, *You keep him in perfect peace whose mind is stayed on You, because he trusts in You.*

"You don't serve Him; He serves you."

Call upon Me in the day of trouble; I will deliver you, and you shall glorify Me (Psalm 50:15).

"You get the help; He gets the glory." Piper

Therefore the LORD waits to be gracious to you, and therefore he exalts Himself to show mercy to you. For the LORD is a God of justice; blessed are all those who wait for Him (Isaiah 30:18). God shows me mercy; then He is exalted. "You get the help; He gets the glory."

I circle back to Acts 17:25: *nor is He served by human hands, as though He needed anything, since He himself gives to all mankind life and breath and everything.* In Piper's example of the Help Wanted sign, he reminds his audience that God isn't worried He won't get His business done if people don't show up. *I am God, and there is no other;*

I am God, and there is none like me, declaring the end from the beginning and from ancient times things not yet done, saying, 'My counsel shall stand, and I will accomplish all my purpose' (Isaiah 46:9-10).

Jesus, God in the flesh, was a living example of our servant Father. Piper turns to Mark 10:41-45: *Whoever would be great among you must be your servant, and whoever would be first among you must be slave of all. For even the Son of Man came to be served but to serve, and to give His life as a ransom for many.*

Like all Jesus' teachings, its upside-down from the world.

Let's go back to Jerry Bridges' observations:

"Our expectation of God's blessing depends on how well we feel we are living the Christian life . . . we innately think so much performance by us earns so much blessing from God . . . .One of the best kept secrets among Christians today is this: *Jesus paid it all. I mean all. He not only purchased your forgiveness of sins and your ticket to heaven, He purchased every blessing and every answer to prayer you will ever receive.*

Again, is there any, even teeny weeny part of you that believes you must earn God's grace? Release it here:

_____

_____

I think about my 'not good enough' mentality. My ongoing compunction to work for God's affection. What an affront to my Father. I hear Him whispering, "Was my Son's sacrifice not enough? You think your deeds add to His settlement? Did He not say, 'It is finished'?"

I must go to the prayer desk, in thanksgiving to Him for exposing this revolutionary truth, and in contrite repentance for thinking I could do anything – *any* thing – to earn His grace.

Whether you are in a season of waiting, or you need to be reminded that you don't work for God, but that He works for you, listen to John Piper's sermon, *God Works for Those Who Wait on Him.* https://www.desiringgod.org/messages/god-works-for-those-who-wait-for-him--2

For additional assurance of God's love, listen to Miss Grace podcast, Smitten. https://www.livewellbygrace.com/speaking-blog/2019/2/4/smitten

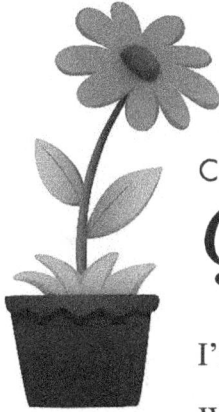

CHAPTER 5
God's Sovereignty

I'm a hypocrite.

With fervor I often pray Psalm 25:4-5. *Make me to know Thy ways, O LORD, teach me Thy paths. Lead me in Thy truth and teach me. For You are the God of my salvation. On You I wait all the day long.*

Then my comfort is compromised and I'm cussing. Same ol' circumstances we've already discussed. Noise. Delays. Inept customer service reps (wasting *my* precious time). Broken systems and stuff.

I'm forced to ask myself, do I believe God is always sovereign? Or honestly, maybe I need to dig deeper and ask, do I believe God's Word?

On the microwave of my vintage mini-motorhome is a sign with a clipart graphic of an RV aside Psalm 32:8,10. *I will instruct thee and teach thee in the ways in which you should go. I will guide thee with mine eyes . . . She who trusts in the Lord shall be surrounded by mercy.*

Then I get stuck in traffic and start disparaging stupid drivers.

Do I just forget God is sovereign, or did I never believe? It seems a critical contemplation. If God is indeed the ultimate authority in *all* things – from long lines to looting – then what's the fuss? He's assured us *all things* work together for good for those who love Him and are called according to His purpose, right? So as much as I shudder to consider, could difficulties be part of my sanctification?

This feels like a notable notion. The key to change. The blanket around my shoulders that assures me of God's promise, "This is unpleasant, but I've allowed it and will use it to bless you." Though I'd love to believe that blessing means meeting a tall, dark, and handsome single man in an irritating long line one day, I have a sneaking suspicion He's referring to the obliteration of my belligerence. I'll take it.

Alistair Begg, with his soothing Scottish accent, has become one of my go-to teachers (http://truthforlife.org). So, when I needed some insights on God's supremacy, I asked Alistair. His sermon entitled "Watchmaker, or All Wise?" fit the bill perfectly.

He started with scriptures declaring God's LORDship. Isaiah 45:6-7 puts it right out there: *I am the Lord, and there is no other. I form light and create darkness; I make well-being and create calamity; I am the Lord, who does all these things.*

Point made; case closed. He is in charge. *I make well-being and create calamity; I am the LORD, who does all these things.*

Psalm 135:6-7 also providentially crossed my path: *Whatever the Lord pleases, he does, in heaven and on earth, in the seas and all deeps. ⁷He it is who makes the clouds rise at the end of the earth, who makes lightnings for the rain and brings forth the wind from his storehouses.* God always stays on point with His messaging.

Has anyone ever told you James 1:2-4 is their favorite passage? Doubt it. *²Count it all joy, my brothers, when you meet trials of various kinds, ³for you know that the testing of your faith produces steadfastness. ⁴And let steadfastness have its full effect, that you may be perfect and complete, lacking in nothing.* Pretty clear: God wants us to celebrate when the going gets tough. Whether He's created the calamity or simply allowed it, it obviously didn't take Him by surprise. Nor is He concerned He's going to lose His right-hand grip on His adopted child. Count it all joy as you remember Isaiah 41:10: *Fear not, for I am with you; be not dismayed, for I am your God; I will strengthen you, I will help you, I will uphold you with my righteous right hand.*

Paul reiterates this message in his letter to the Hebrews: *It is for discipline that you have to endure. God is treating you as sons. For what son is there whom his father does not discipline? If you are left without discipline, in which all have participated, then you are illegitimate children and not sons* (Hebrews 12:7-8).

Alistair hovered awhile over Psalm 107:25-30:

²⁵For he commanded and raised the stormy wind,
    which lifted up the waves of the sea.
²⁶They mounted up to heaven; they went down to the depths;
    their courage melted away in their evil plight;
²⁷they reeled and staggered like drunken men
    and were at their wits' end.
²⁸Then they cried to the LORD in their trouble,
    and he delivered them from their distress.
²⁹He made the storm be still,
    and the waves of the sea were hushed.

[30]Then they were glad that the waters were quiet,
  and he brought them to their desired haven.

It's a familiar sequence. We wander. God stirs up a storm. We cry to Him for help. Waves hush. We rejoice . . . then we wander again. Repeat. Here's the point: I contend I trust God is sovereign, even over the waves of the sea, but I'm not convinced He can hush my neighbor's noise. Could He be doing His work on my side of the fence?

To reinforce the point, Pastor Begg proffered Lamentations 3:37-39: *[37]Who has spoken and it came to pass, unless the Lord has commanded it? [8]Is it not from the mouth of the Most High that good and bad come? [39]Why should a living man complain, a man, about the punishment of his sins?*

If both good and bad come from God, and He commands me to count it all joy when I encounter various trials, assuring me He's doing a good work, who am I to get angry when I don't get my way? How in the world do I have the audacity to complain when, after Jesus' crucifixion and redeeming grace, anything, ANY thing I receive is a bonus blessing.

I'm rattled. Humbled. A bit humiliated. But just in case there was any residual rebellion, Alistair backtracks seven books.

Job got his comeuppance from God in chapters 38-39. His opening statement was, *Who is this that darkens my counsel with words without knowledge?* Ouch! Clearly Job was in for a lashing. And I, too, am instantly crumbled. Job had been crushed by unthinkable heartache, and I'm squawking about bad cell service? (How was it possible people survived for millennia without smart phones?) God's chastising continues for two whole chapters. Take a moment to read the entire passage. It unquestionably clarifies Who's Boss. Here are some highlights:

Who is this that darkens counsel by words without knowledge?. . .
[4]Where were you when I laid the foundation of the earth?. . .

[8]Or who shut in the sea with doors . . .
  [10]and prescribed limits for it
  and set bars and doors,
[11]and said, 'Thus far shall you come, and no farther,
  and here shall your proud waves be stayed'?

[18]Have you comprehended the expanse of the earth?
  Declare, if you know all this.

³⁴*Can you lift up your voice to the clouds,*
    that a flood of waters may cover you?
³⁵*Can you send forth lightnings, that they may go*
    and say to you, 'Here we are'?

³⁹*Can you hunt the prey for the lion,*
    or satisfy the appetite of the young lions,
⁴⁰*when they crouch in their dens*
    or lie in wait in their thicket?
⁴¹*Who provides for the raven its prey,*
    when its young ones cry to God for help,
    and wander about for lack of food?

Chapter 39

¹*Do you know when the mountain goats give birth?*
    Do you observe the calving of the does?
²*Can you number the months that they fulfill,*
    and do you know the time when they give birth,
³*when they crouch, bring forth their offspring,*
    and are delivered of their young?

¹⁹*Do you give the horse his might?*
    Do you clothe his neck with a mane?

²⁶*Is it by your understanding that the hawk soars*
    and spreads his wings toward the south?
²⁷*Is it at your command that the eagle mounts up*
    and makes his nest on high?

God's rhetorical questions are piercing and profound.

He makes His stinging closing argument in Job 40:2: *Shall a faultfinder contend with the Almighty? He who argues with God, let him answer it.*

I shudder.

Who am I to question God's sovereignty?

Has there ever been a time when you questioned God? (Isn't it ironic we can accuse God Almighty of being imprudent?)

Wrestling with God

Jacob was a fighter. Always maneuvering for what he wanted, he was continually in conflict. True to that time, Jacob's name revealed his character. It all started in the womb when he grabbed his twin brother Esau's heel, trying to reach the finish line first. So appropriately, the Hebrew meaning of Jacob is to follow, or to be behind. A second meaning is to supplant (usurp, overthrow, topple), circumvent, assail, or overreach, which was also an accurate typecast. He's regularly referred to as a trickster or schemer. He deceived his dad, Isaac, trying to increase his inheritance by stealing his brother Esau's. He tangled for years with his one-day father-in-law for his daughter's hand in marriage. But one day he finally met his match (Genesis 32).

Jacob had decided to make amends with Esau, but wasn't sure his brother would forgive and forget. Like many successful men, Jacob was good at schmooze. He sent messengers to butter up his brother, offering livestock and servants. His message read, *I have sent to tell my lord, in order that I may find favor in your sight.* The front men returned, telling Jacob that Esau was on his way, accompanied by four hundred soldiers. Not a good sign. Jacob divided his crew in two, so if Esau had ill intent, at least half his people could escape.

Then he started praying, reminding God of His promise. *O God of my father Abraham and God of my father Isaac, O LORD who said to me, 'Return to your country and to your kindred, that I may do you good. I am not worthy of the least of all the deeds of steadfast love and all the faithfulness that you have shown to your servant, for with only my staff I crossed this Jordan, and now I have become two camps. Please deliver me from the hand of my brother, from the hand of Esau, for I fear him, that he may come ad attack me, the mothers with the children. But you said, 'I will surely do you good, and make your offspring as the sand of the sea, which cannot be numbered for multitude.*

His beseeching finished, it was time to bribe. Jacob loaded up his servants with goats, camel, cows, and donkeys and sent them back to Esau to try to talk this thing out. They were instructed to tell him the gifts were from *your servant Jacob. They are a present sent to my lord Esau.* Pretty thick.

While the servants were away, Jacob led his family, household servants, and possessions across the ford of Jabbok, *and Jacob was left alone.*

God does His best work when we've hit bottom and are alone. The story tells of an all-night wrestling match, where God, with just a light touch, dislocated Jacob's hip.

But Jacob was a seasoned fighter. *I will not let you go unless you bless me,* he told his opponent. And at that moment God did bless him, changing his name from "trickster, schemer" to "friends with God."

Several theologians' insights on this passage hit my heart.

Learning through Difficulty

Jacob's all-nighter is one amongst many scriptures that convey a most profound, yet so easily forgotten, Biblical truth: God uses difficult circumstances to get our attention and submission. Jacob was in a pickle. His estranged brother, accompanied by his army, was headed his way. He'd sent his family away, and was left all alone. The king of conniving had played his last card.

I understand planning; it's the entrepreneur's life. My stepfather used to say to me, "Judi, you're selling something nobody wants." And though there were years when employee health promotion was popular, he was right. Eating healthfully and exercising regularly was a hard sell. As a small business owner, growing the cash flow fell solely on my shoulders. Though I regularly *cast all my cares on Him*, I usually took them right back. How many different ways could I reinvent myself? I was reimagining my reimagining. So, Jacob, I get you. Sometimes it feels like calculating and creating is the only option. But . . . that's *self*-reliance. Alistair Begg says, "It's not in human ingenuity but in brokenness and confession that we are transformed and blessed . . . There's nothing wrong with wanting God's blessing. It's about asking and surrendering to receive it, vs. grabbing and/or strategizing." [https://www.truthforlife.org/resources/sermon/he-blessed-him-there/] Sinclair Ferguson imagines God saying, "There must be nothing in your hand but My hand." [*Alone With God*, https://resources.thegospelcoalition.org/library/alone-with-god]

Breaking our Independence

For years I described myself as "independent to a fault," but I didn't really believe the fault part. In fact, like Frank Sinatra I held up my self-reliance as a badge of honor. My feelings didn't stem from the 1970's "I am woman, hear me roar" liberation movement, but rather from the hurt of my history. In my mind I had no help; I was in this battle called life, alone. As a result, I fully related to Jacob's ploys. Since my well-being was completely dependent on my own efforts, everything I did was for my own benefit. Schemer sounds harsh, but most of my moves were to get what I wanted.

After wrestling all night, Jacob had to be tired. At the end of himself. Nigel Beynon observes that with *one touch* God dislocates Jacob's hip. [*Wrestling with God*, https://resources.thegospelcoalition.org/library/wrestling-with-god-en] "Transformation involves tears," he says. God broke Jacob's independent spirit, physically demonstrating, "Sorry son, you're not in charge."

God desires dependence, and calls independence an idol. *Blessed are the meek, for they shall inherit the earth.* Self-sufficiency thwarts God's provision; brokenness begets blessing. For those of us who are survivors, this is a hard lesson. Digging in and fighting hard is in our DNA. We do everything in our power to make life work, because we believe we are our only resource.

Beynon shares the analogy of his 3-year old trying to open a package of biscuits. He's struggling, but insists he can do it himself. When Nigel offers his assistance, he angrily refuses. "No!" He's intent on proving his self-sufficiency, but fails in frustration. Sound familiar?

Stubbornness is infantile.

What areas of your life (situations, concerns, people) do you still try ot manage yourself?

God's Patience

Consider God's patience with Jacob. At any time during the night He could have disappeared, leaving him to fend for himself – bailing on the blessing. But He didn't. He stayed, patiently waiting for Jacob to concede. God *wanted* to bless him.

"Judith, when will you surrender?"

God is waiting for us to ask for His help; He wants to bless us. Remember Pastor Piper's words? "You don't serve Him; He serves you. You get help; He gets the glory."

As the sun was rising, Jacob limped away saying, "My life has been delivered." He had been transformed by grace.

May you, and I, be transformed too. Let's pray:

Lord, You have been patient with my insubordination. How foolish have I been to believe I could well manage my life on my own. Free me from me, Father. Bring me to the end of my plans, ideas and resources. As the beloved song implores, "Make me, Savior, wholly Thine," (All to Jesus I Surrender). May the only thing in my hand be Your hand. Wrestle me empty.

Let's sing together, *I Surrender All*. https://www.youtube.com/watch?v=7x2IpLSfqp8

My angst began to ease with Pastor Alistair's subsequent insight. There seems to be a common confusion: when we find ourselves in a bind, many conclude a loving God would have prevented the problem, so either He's not sovereign, or He's not loving. Precisely my verdict from my financial struggles. "God doesn't love me." But Alistair proposes, "God must have a loving purpose for allowing the circumstance."

Hmmmmm . . . . need to noodle that. Joseph's words to his malicious brothers comes to mind: *What Satan meant for evil, God meant for good* (Genesis 50:20).

Brother Begg then inquires whether we liken God to a watchmaker; He made the universe, and now is sitting back and simply allowing it to run on its own. Is that your view? He's distant? Unengaged? Unconcerned? Let's head back to Job 39. As an animal lover, I find these passages astonishing and heartening.

Do you know when the mountain goats give birth? Do you observe the calving of the does? (vs.1)

Who has let the wild donkey go free? (vs. 5)

Do you give the horse his might? Do you clothe his neck with a mane? (vs. 19)

Is it by your understanding that the hawk soars and spreads his wings toward the south? Is it at your command that the eagle mounts up and makes his nest on high? (vs. 26-27)

God is watching over every minute detail of this grand globe. And shall we review Psalm 139? *You know when I sit down and rise up . . . You discern my thoughts from afar* (ugh . . .) *. . . You search out my path and my lying down and are acquainted with all my ways.* (vs. 2-3)

So back to Alistair's premise: when I'm unhappy with my circumstances, I must remember – assure myself with God's Word – that He allowed it, so it must have a benevolent purpose. Now that's a game-changer, folks.

We think we know.

We think we know what's best for us. What's important. And ironically, what God should do for us.

We think we know.

When have you questioned God regarding your life circumstances; doubted His presence and care?

_____

_____

_____

_____

When was the last time you ate because you were angry? Frustrated? Not getting your way?

_____

_____

_____

_____

Listen to Stirring Words on S.A.N.E. Eating:
https://www.holyhealthclub.com/new-blog/2020/10/28/eating-in-your-right-mind

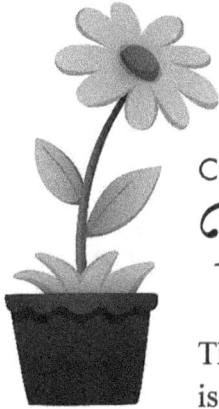

CHAPTER 6
Turn Thou Me

They say continuing to do the same thing and expecting a different result is the definition of insanity. Are you mildly mad?

After acknowledging my anger issues, I tried to exude the fruit of the Spirit by my own efforts, and failed miserably. Can you relate? You've dieted countless times, always with disappointing results. How long will we attempt to sanctify ourselves, instead of relying on the Spirit?

It's time to turn. Change direction. Were you a band member in high school? When the leader called "About face! About face!", the members shouted in response, "1-2-3!", and with perfect choreography the entire troupe faced a different direction. Merriam-Webster defines repent as "to turn from sin." Winnie the Pooh says, "I always get to where I am going by walking away from where I have been."

I was ready to take off judgment, impatience, spitefulness, cussing, and control (well, not sure about control . . .), and put on the fruit of the Spirit, especially peace, patience, gentleness, and kindness. But there was one problem: I was delusional.

Presumably in the context of a guilty conscience vs. literary point of view, I had been reading Psalm 4:2 as if God were speaking. *Oh ye sons of men, how long will ye turn my glory into shame? How long will ye love vanity, and seek after leasing* (lies)? Though it was David who was mourning in this passage, it surely could have been God's words. "Judith, how long will ye turn my glory into shame?" How many people have I decimated with my words, then walked away with zero concern for the carnage? When my anger issues were simply a should, I didn't feel particularly pressured, but *turning God's glory into shame* felt devastating.

Psalm 4:2 is translated in the New International Version, *How long will you love delusions and seek false gods?*

Referring to someone as delusional is rarely a term of endearment. Delusion is defined as "a persistent false psychotic belief." I read that and chuckled. That are me.

Let's untwist the profound phrase, starting with persistent.

persistent – existing for a long time or continuously; incessant, unceasing, unrelenting; remaining infective (infectious) for a relatively long time, as in disease.

Unrelenting means not yielding in determination. Not weakening in vigor, intensity or force.

I can hear Tricia's reference to *besetting* sin. Constantly present or attacking; obsessive. Persistent rises to a whole new level. Anger isn't the anomaly in my life; it's the norm. Common. A regular occurrence. So, check off the first criteria for delusional.

Second, you know you're delusional when you believe something false. Anyone who is convinced he is Alexander the Great, or that he can jump out the 16th floor window and soar into the heavenlies, or that he understands women, would be deemed mentally unstable. A little "affected." Not playing with a full deck. But I am guilty of the same insanity. May I share a few of my fantasies?

- Planes should always be on schedule.
- Customer Service reps should answer the line within three minutes, speak intelligible English, and show genuine concern for my problem.
- Stuff should work. Phones. Computers. Internet. Don't these companies make the big bucks because they make things that work?

These aren't just unrealistic, they're delusional. A fallacy. A fairy tale.

For giggles I consulted Merriam about fairy tale. "A story involving fantastic forces and beings; a story made up, usually designed to *mislead*."

Let's recap. Someone would be considered delusional if she regularly believed something false. Strike two for me and my rants.

The final descriptor for delusional is psychotic. This one makes me a tad nervous, but acknowledgement is the first step toward healing, right?

psychotic – affected or marked by psychosis; mental derangement characterized by defective or lost contact with reality.

I have said and again reiterate: my anger outbursts are like a volcanic eruption, separate from me. They are uncontrollable, and destructive. Though logic might warn me of volatile circumstances and suggest preventative prayer (i.e. plane flights), most often I'm spewing before rationality can take control. Yikes!

But it gets worse.

derangement – to make insane

insane – mentally disordered

"Hi, my name is Judi and I'm mentally disordered."

When I consider my history of temper tantrums, the delusional criteria are complete:

1. It's been happening consistently for a long time.
2. It's built on false beliefs.
3. It makes me insane.

I believe schedules are to be kept, things should work, people should care, and when it doesn't happen, I go mad. Take, for example, the time I was trying to change Internet providers . . .

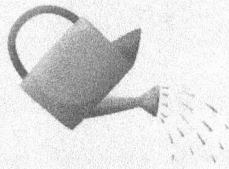

Internet Eruption

"Out in the toolies" might rightly describe my home. Jeff Foxworthy, of you-know-you're-a-redneck fame, once quipped, "You know you're a redneck when you're giving directions to your house and you say, 'then you turn off the paved road . . .'" If the road inconspicuously transitions to dirt, are you still a redneck?

After much research on Internet providers, it became clear I had to settle for satellite. The reception with my first service (term used loosely), when I had it, wasn't too bad. The problem was getting the TV to "find" the satellite. After innumerable calls with the company, all of which ran well beyond my patience quota, still, half the time the picture wouldn't ignite. Have you ever screamed and cussed at an inanimate object? I was done.

The second series of much-too-long calls changed me from one provider to two – one for TV and the other for Internet. Country dwellers swap communications options for serenity. When registering for the Internet piece I had the divine luck of getting a newbie to assist me, who had to put me on hold multiple times to ask his supervisor how to do something. Much to my own surprise, I was pretty patient and empathetic. I asked him no less than three times for confirmation that they did, indeed, service my area. "Yes, I'm looking at the map right now. It's no problem."

He scheduled the installation for the morning of December 24th, just in time for my holiday guests. But when he transferred me to the scheduling department, the second voice said, "I don't know why he would tell you the 24th. We don't have anything available until January 6th."

What could I do? I'd just spent half a year getting the account set up. "OK, schedule me for the 6th." My friends would just have to drive down the hill to find cell reception.

As promised by the TV people, my new satellite arrived the next day, and the tube (Are you old enough to remember that term?) came alive every time I pushed the power button. Wow! Just like the rich folks!

A few days after Christmas I got a call from the Internet company: "We've mistakenly overbooked on January 6th. We need to move you to the 10th." Are you serious? I was originally told three days, which went to two weeks, that now is turning into nearly three weeks with no Internet. I was quite clear about my dissatisfaction – how greatly they'd inconvenienced me – "your incompetence is beyond comprehension" – all directed at a minimum wage scheduler who had absolutely nothing to do with the previous bumblings, nor did she really care about my hardships. All I could do was wait and consider it patience practice.

When the white van pulled into my driveway the anticipated installation morning, I ran out to meet him, doing the happy dance. "I'm so excited to see you! I haven't had Internet for three weeks!"

He wasn't happying with me. "I don't know why they sent me out here. We don't service this area."

My brain took a moment to comprehend his words. What? "Are you kidding? I asked the guy three times to confirm they came out this far and he assured me they do."

"They don't know. They're just order takers."

Are you delusional too? Do your eating episodes usually include the 3D?

1. They've been happening consistently for a long time.
2. They're built on false beliefs.
3. They make you insane.

Maybe it's time to turn.

Turn Thou Me

I knew I wasn't able to transform my heart on my own, but I had a hopeful insight from Jeremiah 31:18: *Turn Thou me, and I shall be turned; for Thou art the LORD my God.*

Remember David Powlison's words of wisdom: "Self-manufactured changes do not dislodge almighty me from the center of my tiny self-manufactured universe." [*Seeing with New Eyes*]

Deuteronomy 30:6 says *And the LORD your God will circumcise your heart and the heart of your offspring, so that you will love the LORD your God with all your heart and with all your soul, that you may live.* Note Who's the surgeon, and who's the patient.

I began to pray every day:

Turn Thou me, Lord.
Turn Thou me.
Please Lord, turn me.
For then I shalt be turned, for You are my God.

I wanted to turn from anger to grace; from anxiety to peace.

What about you? As you seek to establish new health habits, what do you want to turn from, and to? Consider overcoming:

- Satan's lies
- Cravings
- Temptation
- Fleshly desires
- Darkness
- Fear
- Temporal satisfaction
- The world

- Folly
- Guilt
- Shame
- Unbelief

Oh, the joy of putting all that mess in the rear-view mirror! Instead focus on:

- God's Word
- God's promises
- God's provision
- God's power
- The Good Shephard
- Belief
- Faith
- Wisdom
- Light

Do some writing about what you want to turn from/to, and why.

_____

_____

_____

Exercise is a perfect example. When you ask people to share what comes to mind when they consider it, you hear things like painful, hard, time consuming, inconvenient and sweaty. What if you reframed the endeavor, considering it a nurturing time of self-care and stress relief? Or step it up a notch and refer to your walks as Worship Workouts™, a sacred escape with your Father when you memorize His Word and/or sing songs of praise. Which activity captivates you?

The new view brings a breath of fresh air, both literally and figuratively. Take some time to go before your Father, asking Him to turn you in a new direction.

Confession

Turning starts with confession.

We humans are quite reluctant to admit our wrongdoing. We think we're pretty good chaps, and don't quickly see our willful ways. Let's revisit Alistair Begg's statement:

"When I'm unhappy with my circumstances, I must remember that He allowed it, so it must have a benevolent purpose."

Judi's translation: When I get angry, I'm saying God isn't sovereign, or He isn't good.

Gulp.

It was a true statement that I was forced to honestly consider.

As I said in the chapter on God's Sovereignty, I'm a hypocrite. I believe God is in control when life is rolling my way, but when I hit a bump, I assume He's gone AWOL. Just like Job I wail: *God has cast me into the mire, and I have become like dust and ashes. I cry to you for help and you do not answer me; I stand, and you only look at me. You have turned cruel to me;* (Job 30:19-21).

Oh, the drama.

Our turning verse from Jeremiah was prefaced by Israel's regret. It was written in the context of Ephraim (Israel) grieving yet again over her waywardness, "like an untrained calf." She's bemoaning her self-induced exile, clearly revealing her inability to change on her own accord. Their "self-reformation," as David Powlison called it, wasn't working, so she's begging the LORD to turn her.

Psalm 51 offers an excellent guideline for confession. David was on his knees in contrite repentance, begging God for forgiveness and change. Here are some highlights:

Have mercy on me, O God, according to your steadfast love; according to your abundant mercy blot out my transgressions. ²Wash me thoroughly from my iniquity, and cleanse me from my sin! ³For I know my transgressions, and my sin is ever before me. ⁴Against you, you only, have I sinned and done what is evil in your sight, so that you may be justified in your words and blameless in your judgment . . . ¹⁶For you will not delight in sacrifice, or I would give it; you will not be pleased with a burnt offering. ¹⁷The sacrifices of God are a broken spirit; a broken and contrite heart, O God, you will not despise.

Have you ever prayed this scripture in an attempt to express your heartfelt remorse for deeds done or left undone? When there is profound sorrow after sin, you know you are being sanctified.

Regret begets repentance. Synonyms include remorse, sorrow, and lament. Only after we feel sincere contrition will we turn. Though it took a while, I finally came to the place of genuine grief over my unbridled rancor. I hated how I felt afterward. Like Peter at the third crowing of the cock, I was devastated by disappointing my Lord.

Has over-indulging ever left you feeling the same way? Reminisce.

_____

_____

_____

Few relish confession. We must remember, God is slow to anger and abounding in steadfast love. The Holy Spirit is our Helper, *not* our drill sergeant. Confession seems to suggest we did something wrong. "Lord forgive me for my cranky spirit." But maybe more importantly, it's admitting our weakness. Our brokenness. Our inability to do what's right, even when we try earnestly. Consider calling out to your Father, not in shame but in need. David prayed, *Create in me a clean heart, O God; renew a right spirit within me* (Psalm 51:10). Go to the God of unbounding grace with an open, honest, contrite spirit. Admit not only your poor choices but your wounded heart. Proverbs 28:13 reiterates our assurance of mercy: *Whoever conceals his transgressions will not prosper, but he who confesses and forsakes them will obtain mercy.*

Meditate on the verses below and see if they don't ease your angst over honest admission. As always, I've left writing space.

But who can discern their own errors? Forgive my hidden faults. [13]*Keep your servant also from willful sins; may they not rule over me. Then I will be blameless, innocent of great transgression. May these words of my mouth and this meditation of my heart be pleasing in your sight, Lord, my Rock and my Redeemer* (Psalm 19:12-14, NASB).

The sacrifices of God are a broken spirit; a broken and contrite heart, O God, you will not despise (Psalm 51:17).

_____

_____

_____

Extra credit: Read Psalm 88. Aaahhh . . . .

Miss Grace would like to offer a little commentary on turning, using Jonah as her example.

https://www.livewellbygrace.com/speaking-blog/2019/5/6/jonah

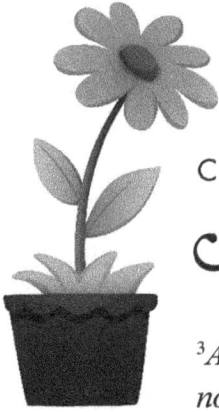

CHAPTER 7
A New Heart

³And you show that you are a letter from Christ delivered by us, written not with ink but with the Spirit of the living God, not on tablets of stone but on tablets of human hearts (2 Corinthians 3:3).

I knew in my own strength I couldn't play nice. When that volcano of anger started to rumble, all self-control vanished. I didn't need a pocket full of anger management tips; I needed a new heart. The good news is God specializes in heart transplants.

It has always amazed me that when I'm earnestly seeking the Lord's counsel, scriptures appear. How in the world did I land in Ezekiel? It spoke plainly and directly: *²⁵I will sprinkle clean water on you, and you shall be clean from all your uncleannesses, and from all your idols I will cleanse you. ²⁶And I will give you a new heart, and a new spirit I will put within you. And I will remove the heart of stone from your flesh and give you a heart of flesh. ²⁷And I will put my Spirit within you, and cause you to walk in my statutes and be careful to obey my rules* (Ezekiel 36:25-27).

I was stunned. I clutched my Lord's promise like Linus his blanket. I read and reread it multiple times a day. Stuck it in my pocket so I could claim it while I was out walking. I personalized and prayed it regularly. "Lord, sprinkle me with Your clean water."

It seems to me that our heart health is God's highest priority; it is the crux of Jesus' sacrifice at Calvary. We know that we *all have sinned and fall short of the glory of God* (Romans 3:23). And Jeremiah 17:9 says, *The heart is deceitful above all things, and desperately sick; who can understand it?* Then Matthew 5:18-20 blatantly states: *¹⁸But what comes out of the mouth proceeds from the heart, and this defiles a person. ¹⁹For out of the heart come evil thoughts, murder, adultery, sexual immorality, theft, false witness, slander. ²⁰These are what defile a person.* I was Exhibit A.

But God was promising to give me a kinder, gentler model. He promised to remove my heart of stone and give me a soft, heart of flesh. "Bring it!", I cheered.

Wouldn't it be great if changing our thinking and our actions was as simple as editing a Word document? Highlight – delete – done. Unfortunately, that's not God's way. Just like we value what we pay for, we value that which we've labored with the Lord. Consider an athlete in training; s/he rigorously works day after day, months on end, to hone her/his skills. Sacrifice and discipline are required to win. As Hebrews 12:11 says, *For the moment all discipline seems painful rather than pleasant, but later it yields the peaceful fruit of righteousness to those who have been trained by it.* I had a sneaking suspicion my new heart wasn't going to be delivered as quickly as Amazon Prime.

Sanctification is slow. Remember David Platt's words? "Sanctification is a lifelong process of growing in Christ-likeness." For all you Type-A's like me, strap in for the long haul. As they say, this is a marathon, not a sprint.

So how do I know if my new heart is en route?

Faith. *The righteous shall live by faith* (Romans 1:17). *Blessed are those who have not seen and yet have believed* (John 20:29).

Back to Paul Tripp: "It is important to remember the new character qualities and behavior patterns that are in your life because of Jesus. You already have a new heart. You have been radically changed by his grace and are being progressively restored day by day. That is the focus of God's work in your life right now. [*How People Change*, Paul Tripp, p. 117]

It reminds me of 2 Corinthians 3:18. [18]*And we all, with unveiled face, beholding the glory of the Lord are being transformed into the same image from one degree of glory to another. For this comes from the Lord who is the Spirit.*

Being transformed . . . from one degree of glory to another.

" . . . progressively restored day by day."

This is a confusing paradigm that Tricia calls Now, and Not Yet.

- God has changed us, but we're still imperfect.
- The Holy Spirit lives inside us, and our snitty self-centeredness can still surface.
- We have been cleansed, but are still dirty, but God sees us and is making us clean.

It's a mind-bender, but *the righteous shall live by faith.* I continued to pray Ezekiel 36:25-27.

Gracious, merciful Father,

I confess I am unclean. My thoughts, words, and heart are filthy before You. I am idol-ridden. It's all about almighty me. My way. My time. My comfort.

If it be Thy will, O LORD, sprinkle me anew with Your clean water. Make me clean from all my uncleanness. Pry me from my idols. Fill me with worship vs. self-absorption. Cleanse me from willfulness. Remind me You are sovereign in all things, even circumstances I don't understand, agree with, or like. Create in me a clean heart, Father, one that loves – seeks to listen and understand vs. judge and condemn. Open my eyes to see as You see. To listen as You listen. To care like you care. Remove my heart of stone – rigid, angry, closed, unyielding – and give me a soft, open, fully alive, compassionate, heart. Help me to hear Your Holy Spirit within me. Protect me from Satan's entrenched lies. Reveal Your ways. Transform me with Your truth. Thy Word is truth. Cause me – make me – move me to walk in Your statutes. May I be careful, cautious, acutely aware, to obey Your rules, follow Your commands, walk in Your Spirit. May I ever remember the letter killeth, but Your Spirit giveth life.

May my heart be ever athirst for Thee.

Amen

Make Me

"Make me!"

Remember, as kids, shouting that dare to a sibling or other foe? "You can't make me!"

There's One Who *can* make us, praise Him for that.

As I said earlier, when I am seeking God's direction, one of my favorite passages is Psalm 25:4-5: *Make me to know Thy ways, O LORD; teach me Thy paths. Lead me in Thy truth and teach me. For you are the God of my salvation; on You I wait all the day long.*

Notice it begins with *make me.* Cause me. Produce in me. I'm not the Maker; I'm the makee. That's a critical concept in turning. Turn Thou me. Make me. I've tried to make myself, and failed. Make me, Lord.

Paul's prayer to the church in Thessalonica in 2 Thessalonians 1:11-12 was that *God would make them* worthy of His calling. That He would fulfill every resolve for good and every work of faith *by His power.* Again, God's making; we are being made.

I have a tendency to think God's sole concern is my sanctification, and certainly He wants us to grow in our Christ-likeness. But notice a few more make me's:

You make me to lie down in green pastures (Psalm 23:2). For someone who struggles with the Drill Sergeant Dad, making me lie down in a nurturing place doesn't quite fit. While I'm out in the world, sweating to be good enough, He's calling me – making me if I would allow – to safe places. Similarly, Psalm 4:8 says *You make me dwell in safety.* My tendency is to drift toward danger, but He steers me back to His protected pasture. "The safest place to be is surrendered to God," says Charles Stanley. [In Touch Ministries, intouch.org]

He makes me. Praise God.

Musing on God purposely leading me toward comfort, care, and security shook my stony heart. Safety had been my life's pursuit. He makes me lie down in green pastures, not stand outside in the rain. He makes me dwell His sanctuary, when I can easily wander into treacherous situations. He makes me worthy of His calling, knowing I'm not on my own accord. He makes me dwell in a more comfortable place. So why am I fighting Him?

Tricia and I had been discussing Ephesians 4 where Paul talks about taking off/putting on. I was clear on the concept of taking off contempt and putting on politeness, but again, I couldn't "Just do it" as Nike suggests. Rather than hovering long on taking off anger, we began focusing on what I was to put on. To my surprise, it wasn't kindness. It was Jesus. Remember David Platt's sermon* we considered back when we were embracing grace? Here's another compelling quote from that message: "Where we focus our minds comes out in our lives. The more we look to Christ, the more we'll look like Christ."

I could easily have done a character study on Jesus and found the traits I wanted to emulate, but Tricia in her not-so-subtle manner used the analogy of kingdom building. When I found myself wanting to rant, she challenged me to ask, "Who's kingdom am I building right now? The kingdom of God, or of Judi?"

Dang.

---

* https://radical.net/sermon/the-cross-and-christian-sanctification/

Then she provided a graphic, called The Y Diagram, that pretty much slammed me:

GOD   SELF

GOD	SELF
Psalm 95:6-9	Judges 17:6
Deuteronomy 6:17-19	Proverbs 13:15

TRIAL

When trials come, what rules your heart, your fiery desires, or God's commands? Whose kingdom are you building? There are only two options: the God-centered life, or the self-centered life. Temptations and turmoil reveal which way we lean.

Consider the last time you experienced internal conflict over exercising. (Yesterday?) Jot your thoughts below. Does the banter reveal the battle?

_____

_____

As I walked through this process, after uplifting time in the Word, feeling my heart had been stirred, I would tumble in despair when yet again, I nipped at someone for their oversight in placating me. Do you get discouraged when you not only haven't reached your goal, you can't even see the finish line? Take a moment to acknowledge the small steps of progress you have made in the last few weeks. Remember, o*ne degree of glory to another . . .*

_____

_____

Next read Philippians 1:6: *He who began a good work in you will complete it until the day of Christ Jesus.* Say aloud five times: "He who began a good work in me will complete it until the day of Christ."

Do you feel refreshed? Released? Unburdened? Oh, the joy of coming before a merciful Father. Now it's time to celebrate. Stand up a moment and listen to Carrie Underwood sing Jesus Take the Wheel. Sing it like you mean it! https://www.youtube.com/watch?v=k_OpRlUZQoI

"Jesus take the wheel. Take it from my hands, 'cuz I can't do it on my own . . ." Is there a specific circumstance where you can sing that lyric with earnestness?

_____

_____

What outcome can we expect when we surrender? Let's return to the Word.

Surrender stimulates hope.

You're sitting on the side of the road with a flat tire. It's getting dark and there's no way you can change it yourself. You're away from home, know no one in the area, and don't have A.A.A. How would you feel?

_____

_____

But if you do have A.A.A., how would you feel?

_____

_____

At the risk of sounding sacrilegious, God is the ultimate A.A.A. In all of life's challenges that you have absolutely no ability to tackle on your own, as His child He is always a prayer away. I love Ephesians 1:19: *That you may know the hope to which He has called you . . . and what is the immeasurable greatness of His power toward us who believe.*

Consider the key words and add your thoughts:

immeasurable – boundless, immense, enormous

power – ability to do, capacity to act, authority, influence

His boundless capacity to act. His enormous influence. His immense ability to do for you.

But . . . . you gotta believe. You must acknowledge you can't, but He can. There's no question: Sincere surrender to the power of the Almighty stirs grand hope.

Consider the following and note any insight for your food and fitness ambitions:

Humble thyself, therefore, under the mighty hand of God and he will lift you up in due time (1 Peter 5:6).

May the God of hope fill you with all joy and peace in believing, so that by the power of the Holy Spirit you may abound in hope (Romans 15:13).

Do these stir up optimism? Why or why not?

_____

_____

I get it. Even with all these compelling scriptures, hope can be elusive. You can't muster confidence. Faith is faint. Remember, faith isn't about trying, it's about trusting. Go back to the War Room. Confess your doubts. Pray aloud: "Father, I yearn for the joy and peace of believing in the strength of surrendering to You. I want to trust You like a child – to have the faith of a tiny mustard seed. Holy Spirit, come upon me that I might abound in hope."

Then go for a walk in one of your favorite places.

Surrender provides strength.

At the risk of being redundant, remember David Powlison's words about the sabotage of self-reliance. "No one can truly change who does not know and rely on gifts from the hand of the Lord . . . Self-manufactured changes do not dislodge almighty me from the center of my tiny self-manufactured universe." [David Powlison, *Seeing With New Eyes* p. 48]

Almighty me certainly is stubborn! Even though you've flailed and failed through your own efforts – "willpower" – somehow, like the little train, you still think you can. Guess what gang, you can't. You've proven that. It's time to let go and let God. His power is perfected in your weakness.

How do the following verses relate to your physical care efforts?

God opposes the proud but gives grace to the humble. ⁷Submit yourselves therefore to God. Resist the devil, and he will flee from you (James 4:6-7).

To you, O Lord, I call; my rock, be not deaf to me, lest, if you be silent to me, I become like those who go down to the pit. ²Hear the voice of my pleas for mercy, when I cry to you for help, when I lift up my hands toward your most holy sanctuary (Psalm 28:1-2).

Are you ready to surrender? To lay your burden down? To let Jesus take the wheel? Take a moment to write him a letter, sharing your softened heart. Write Him a letter, sharing your softened heart.

_____

_____

_____

_____

_____

_____

_____

_____

Before we move on, let's be sure that you're sure you've cast all your cares on Him (1 Peter 5:7). You want to be certain that backpack of concerns you habitually clutch is empty. Grab any stowaway worries and with both hands, lift your arms and your eyes to the heavens, and thank God that He wants to carry your load . . . ALL your load. Hold your arms high until you can hold them no longer. Release and relax, feeling the strength and freedom of a surrendered sheep.

The Final Result: Freedom

Americans are a blessed people. We think freedom is the norm and a right, when in fact, many around the globe are imprisoned. Unfortunately, here in the U.S. we often incarcerate ourselves. We overspend and pile on too much debt. Alcohol or drugs strangle us. Even our thoughts, when we believe Satan's lies, become a dungeon of gloom. But God . . .

After moving to the Pacific Northwest, Halloween always marked the start of my journey to sunnier, dryer climates. One year however, God's still small voice (via two root canals and RV issues) said, "My plan is for you to stay home this winter." I'm embarrassed to admit, I bellyached nearly non-stop over the dreary days. But one day I had an epiphany. After seeing the hourly rain report it became clear there would be no breaks, so Boaz (my sweet Rottie-mix) and I were going have to endure a wet walk.

So, we did.

And we didn't die.

As I was wandering in the woods getting sprinkled, the revelation dawned: I'd been reacting. Dark clouds triggered dark moods. I wasn't getting my way (crisp temps and pristine blue sky), so I'd pout. Or grumble. Or both. I was allowing the storms outside to stir up storms inside. Over what? Muddy boots? Really? For someone who relishes her freedom, it was clear I was imprisoning myself. My self-centered chatter was holding my joy captive. Dumb. So instead of reacting to rain (or traffic or unexpected expenses or . . .) I decided I'd start FREE-acting. Jesus said, *"Truly, truly, I say to you, everyone who practices sin is a slave to sin. ³⁵The slave does not remain in the house forever; the son remains forever. ³⁶So if the Son sets you free, you will be free indeed* (John 8:34-36).

The more fully and consistently you embrace God's goodness, grace, wisdom and sovereignty, the more freedom you will experience, spiritually, emotionally and physically. Consider how 2 Corinthians 3:17 describes your physical victory. *Now the Lord is the Spirit, and where the Spirit of the Lord is, there is freedom.*

How can you start FREE-acting instead of reacting? What scriptures will propel your decision?

_____

_____

_____

_____

_____

_____

_____

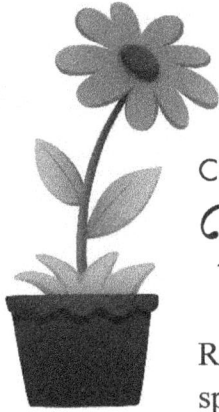

CHAPTER 8
Behold Him

Remember John MacArthur's prod to practice our position? What is the spiritual quarterback's training regimen? Now that we've admitted we can't sanctify ourselves, how do we train for godliness? Let's defer to a couple of those to whom John Piper fondly refers as "dead saints."

John Milton, in his renowned poem, *Paradise Lost*, said, "The mind is its own place, and in itself can make heaven of hell, and hell of heaven." When I'm spinning in a rage, my mind has turned my life into hell. When you are obsessed by something sweet, you feel overpowered by it. But God's holy Spirit through His holy Word refocuses our thoughts.

Thomas Chalmers was a 19th century Scottish preacher whose most famous work was entitled, *The Expulsive Power of a New Affection*. It was based on 1 John 2:15: *Do not love the world or the things in the world. If anyone loves the world, the love of the Father is not in him.* Chalmers' basic premise was the only way to defeat a worldly longing is to replace it with affection for God. He writes, "It is seldom that any of our tastes are made to disappear by a mere process of natural extinction . . . .The heart must have something to cling to – and never by its own voluntary consent will it so denude itself of all its attachments . . . .In a word, if the way to disengage the heart from the positive love of one great an ascendant object, is to fasten it in positive love to another, then it is not by exposing the worthlessness of the former, but by addressing to the mental eye the worth and excellence of the latter, that all old things are to be done away and all things are to become new . . . We know of no other way by which to keep the love of the world out of our heart, than to keep in our hearts the love of God – and no other way by which to keep our hearts in love of God, than building ourselves up on our most holy faith."

Whew. That was a brain-bender. Let's unwrap it.

"It is seldom that any of our tastes are made to disappear by a mere process of natural extinction." Surely Pastor Chalmers wasn't giving a weight loss pep-talk, but the truth remains: You're not going to stop eating tempting foods by "natural extinction." "Just do it," is a fantasy. We won't, because we can't. We can only change our affections when we "disengage the heart from the positive love of one great an ascendant object," and "fasten it in positive love to another." This was exactly Paul's message to the Ephesian church: . . . *put off your old self, which belongs to your former manner of life and is corrupt through deceitful desires, and to be renewed in the spirit of your minds, and to put on the new self, created after the likeness of God in true righteousness and holiness* (Ephesians 4:22-24).

Therein lies your three-step process of transformation:

1. Put off the old self. Identify those people, places, foods, habits, that are unhelpful, and commit to turn from them.
2. Be renewed in your mind. Identify specific scriptures you will claim for strength in sustaining your new path. Memorize 2 Peter 1:3. *His divine power has granted to us all things that pertain to life and godliness, through the knowledge of Him.*
3. Put on the new self. This is the work of godly self-control in partnership with the Holy Spirit, transforming you through His holy Word. Remember 2 Timothy 3:16-17: *All Scripture is breathed out by God and profitable for teaching, for reproof, for correction, and for training in righteousness, that the man of God may be complete, equipped for every good work.*

Jude 20-21 reads: [20]*But you, beloved, building yourselves up in your most holy faith and praying in the Holy Spirit,* [21]*keep yourselves in the love of God, waiting for the mercy of our Lord Jesus Christ that leads to eternal life.* Desires of the flesh won't just magically disappear – they must be overpowered by keeping ourselves in the love of God. How do we do that? By praying, reading His Word, worshipping, and engaging in community.

Put on God's Word

"There is a relationship between being filled with the Spirit, and being filled with the Word of God." [Sinclair Ferguson, *Can I Ever Be Happy?*, sermon on Psalm 1, https://resources.thegospelcoalition.org/library/can-i-ever-be-happy]

Beyond family and friends, do you follow folks on Facebook and Twitter? What value does that time and attention give you? If Jesus was tweeting today, would you be following Him? Why or why not?

_____

_____

_____

The Bible is God-breathed (2 Timothy 3:16). According to 2 Peter, *men spoke from God as they were carried along by the Holy Spirit* (2 Peter 1:20-21). So scripture isn't simply ancient commentary. It's God speaking directly to His children, and He's not limited to 280 characters. Again, the Word is *profitable for teaching, for reproof, for correction, and for training in righteousness, that the man of God may be complete, equipped for every good work* (2 Timothy 3:16-17). This spoke directly to me on my anger. Stepping up for reproof and correction was a bit intimidating, but I was drawn to being *equipped for every good work*. As I've mentioned multiple times, I was confident I was incompetent when it came to managing my mouth. I knew I needed training in righteousness. Wouldn't you like to be equipped for the good work of self-care?

Titus 2:11-12 reads: *For the grace of God has appeared, bringing salvation for all people, training us to renounce ungodliness and worldly passions, and to live self-controlled, upright, and godly lives in the present age.*

train: to develop or form the habits, thoughts, or behavior of a person by discipline and instruction; to make proficient by instruction and practice

God will help us develop new habits, thoughts, or behaviors by discipline and instruction. How exactly does He do that? Let's re-read 2 Peter 1:3 and add verse 4: *His divine power has granted to us all things that pertain to life and godliness, through the knowledge of Him who called us to his own glory and excellence, by which He has granted to us His precious and very great promises, so that through them you may become partakers of the divine nature, having escaped from the corruption that is in the world because of sinful desire.*

It always helps to consider scripture from all angles. Let's read this passage backwards:

We can *participate in God's divine nature*.

participate: to take or have a part, as with others

partake: to share; to receive, take, or have a share of

Like mine, your brain may be debating, "Me? A Divine nature? Surely you jest." Let's consider some of the attributes of God's divine nature: Gracious and merciful, slow to anger, abounding in steadfast love (Psalm 145:8). Always exuding love, joy, peace, patience, kindness, goodness, faithfulness, gentleness, and self-control (Galatians 5:22-23). I don't know about you, but so far, I'm not seeing a resemblance. So how can we better live out His divine nature?

Through His precious and very great promises. Through the knowledge of Him, revealed in His Word. Specifically, what promises are you claiming so you can be a partaker of His divine nature?

_____

_____

Through the knowledge of Him, revealed in His word. If we are to become His image-bearers, it is imperative we know Him. To know Him is to love Him, and to love Him is to know Him. How might you get better acquainted with God, and request He direct and energize your fitness efforts?

_____

_____

Granting us all things that pertain to life and godliness. Graciousness. Kindness. Self-control.

Remember what John said in chapter 15 of his letter? Take a moment to read the first half. *"Apart from me ye can do nothing."* But *His divine power has granted to us all things that pertain to life and godliness,*

Let's step back and review:

1. Through God's power (not ours)
2. As we claim His promises (meditating on His Word)
3. We will share His divine nature (through progressive transformation)
4. To live a godly, self-controlled life. (Victory!)

Now let's consider each phrase and how it can help us in our process of change. I'll start, you follow.

[3]*His divine power has granted to us all things that pertain to life and godliness,*

Me: His power has granted, (imparted, provided, supplied) all I need, including patience and meekness, to be godly. i.e. considerate and pleasant in all circumstances.

You: _____

_____

_____

through the knowledge of him who called us to his own glory and excellence,

Me: Two things. 1. I need to know Him – "experience Him" as JI Packer suggests in *Knowing God,* and 2. I'm called to emulate His glory and excellence, and that's not happening when I'm blowing a gasket.

You: _____

_____

_____

so that through them you may become partakers of the divine nature, having escaped from the corruption that is in the world because of sinful desire.

Me: By clinging to His promises my heart is changed. I share His divine nature. I escape the corruption of bowing to the kingdom of Judi.

You: _____

_____

_____

That's some powerful preachin', Paul!

When I am walking in the flesh, I am forgetting God is sovereign, has a divine plan, and will provide me everything I need. By claiming His promises, I will share in His nature, living a godly, self-controlled life.

Luke 4:1-2 always makes me giggle. *And Jesus, full of the Holy Spirit, returned from the Jordan and was led by the Spirit in the wilderness for forty days, being tempted by the devil. And he ate nothing during those days. And when they were ended, he was hungry.* Hmmm . . . hungry after nearly six weeks. Quite the understatement, Dr. Luke. True to character, Satan tried to capitalize on Jesus' weakness, challenging His power, authority, and sovereignty when He had low blood sugar. Sound familiar? But did you notice? He retaliated with the Word. He destroyed Satan's lies with Truth. So, when your defenses are down, be prepared to combat Satan with scripture.

Jesus didn't just read the Word, He *knew* the Word. He was filled with the Word. Psalm 1 describes the man whose *delight is in the law of the LORD, and on His law he meditates day and night. He is like a tree planted by streams of water that yields its fruit in its season, and its leaf does not wither, and in all that he does, he prospers.* Are you ready to be both spiritually and physically fruitful and prosperous? Delight yourself in the Word, meditating on it day and night. True transformation requires not just reading scripture, but ingesting it. Memorizing it. Pastor John Piper says "If you don't have strong word in your heart and your mind . . . .putting itself forward and stored up in your memory, you'll be a pushover for the devil and your own flesh . . . .meditation means reading it, memorizing it, chewing on it, meditating on it, pondering it, thinking about it until you see it the way God wants it to be seen, namely as infinitely precious and satisfying, and then it changes everything . . . ." [*http://www.desiringgod.com; *Hold Fast to the Word and Pray for Us*, based on 2 Thessalonians 2:13-3:5]

Isn't that what you want? To be permanently changed, done being a pushover for the devil and those darned disordered desires? Then saturate your mind in God's Word.

Miss Grace shares her secret to successful scripture memory here: https://www.livewell-bygrace.com/speaking-blog/2018/10/16/a-grand-bargain

Read the passages below and decide which one (or two . . .) you will memorize to throw at Satan next time he tries to trip you up.

Philippians 4:13
Isaiah 40:29-31
2 Corinthians 12:9-10
Psalm 28:7-8

I love Psalm 22:19. *But you, O LORD, do not be far off! O you my help, come quickly to my aid!* Keep that one in your pocket!

Now go to YouTube and sing *Thy Word* with the Mullett family:
https://www.youtube.com/watch?v=Afz0q0cQjlI&feature=youtu.be

If you don't know *Thy Word* by heart, at minimum memorize the first verse and the chorus so any time you are tempted to make a destructive choice you can sing yourself back to sanity, right in Satan's face.

When I feel afraid,
And think I've lost my way
Still, you're there right beside me
Nothing will I fear
As long as you are near
Please be near me to the end

Thy Word is a lamp unto my feet and a light unto my path.
Thy Word is a lamp unto my feet and a light unto my path.

Beware of Bully Brain

Is your brain a bully? You start your day by setting your sights on self-control, but before your oatmeal's been digested, you walk into the break room to refresh your coffee and the mental torment starts: "That custard-filled croissant sure looks good . . . ." And it's relentless. After work you hear yourself say, "I don't feel like walking tonight. . . ." Then after a tough week you think, "I deserve it . . ." Maybe your personal script is pride, fear or shame. Or like me, you are the contentious critic. Do defeat and doubt get high scores, because you're convinced you're a failure? Welcome to Satan's seduction. Remember, he's hard at work to kill, steal and destroy you. The only way to battle his baloney is with truth. But just like our biceps aren't going to get any stronger unless we consistently stress them, so spiritual strength requires regular training. Reading and memorizing the Word of God transforms our thoughts which alters our actions. David Powlison says, "You cannot destroy the tumult of self-will by sheer will . . . The only way you can wrestle yourself down (from self-will) is by the promises of God. You need help the way a drowning man needs help from outside himself to rescue him." [*Seeing With New Eyes*, p. 81] The Word is sharper than a two-edged sword, smashing seductive thoughts. Just like you highlight and paste to replace errant text in a Word document, you must practice overwriting destructive yearnings with God's promises of strength through the Spirit. How does the passage below pertain to your commitment to self-care?

I appeal to you therefore, brothers, by the mercies of God, to present your bodies as a living sacrifice, holy and acceptable to God, which is your spiritual worship. Do not be conformed to this world, but be transformed by the renewal of your mind, that by testing you may discern what is the will of God, what is good and acceptable and perfect (Romans 12:1-2).

be transformed by the renewal of your mind, . . . In one short phrase, eight simple words, the nearly $70 billion diet industry is debunked. Much to program peddler's chagrin, it's not about purging your pantry or tracking your steps. True transformation comes only by renewing your mind, and the only trustworthy truth is the Word of God.

Before we mull over more scriptures, take a moment to consider your inner chatter about your physical condition and appearance. Are your thoughts helping or hindering you? Would you ever be so unkind to anyone else?

_____

_____

Back to the Book:

Abide in me, and I in you. As the branch cannot bear fruit by itself, unless it abides in the vine, neither can you, unless you abide in me. I am the vine; you are the branches. Whoever abides in me and I in him, he it is that bears much fruit. For apart from me ye can do nothing (John 15:4-5).

Ah ha! The secret to bashing your bully brain is abiding in the Vine. Abide is defined by Merriam Webster as "to wait for; await; to endure without yielding; withstand; to bear patiently; to remain stable or fixed in state; to conform to; to acquiesce in." Let's consider the classic post-supper scene. You're not really hungry, but more accurately, bored. Or agitated. ("That bum . . .") Or maybe lonely. There's one more serving of mint chocolate chip in the freezer. (What happened to the rest of the gallon?) "Sure would taste good . . ." How's the vine-abiding going in that moment?

Do you have a hungry heart? Miss Grace would love to love on you. https://www.livewellbygrace.com/speaking-blog/2019/6/24/hungry-heart

Sometimes it seems our spirit-filling fades away. Does the Spirit come-and-go like a typical teenager? No, He's always there to help. It's our fickle brain that changes. You're filled with the love of Jesus during your morning quiet time, but you'd prefer to be filled by the sweetness of sugar after lunch. It's all about taking every thought captive. When temptation tries to distract and derail you, overpower it with the Word. It's sort of like when you're sitting out in your garden relishing a peaceful moment, do you choose to focus on the birds' serenade, or the neighbor's lawnmower? The world is loud. Hearing His still, small voice requires intentional attention. When you are tempted to do or not do your intended temple care, are you abiding? Or are you listening to the lawnmower? Coach yourself here on how next time you will redirect your listening:

_____

_____

_____

If then you have been raised with Christ, seek the things that are above, where Christ is, seated at the right hand of God. ²Set your minds on things that are above, not on things that are on earth (Colossians 3:1-2).

Consider a typical day. On average, how many times do you think about eating, especially dreaming of unhealthy foods? When you think about your evening walk, is it with enthusiastic anticipation or drudgery? Be honest.

_____

_____

_____

Why do you give food so much bandwidth? What does it represent to you? What emotions arise when you envision eating your favorite foods? Take a deep breath. This could stir up some dirt.

_____

_____

_____

Kim Taylor shares how she overcame her emotional attachment to sugar here: https://www.holyhealthclub.com/new-blog/2020/6/24/using-sugar-to-soothe

This Book of the Law shall not depart from your mouth, but you shall meditate on it day and night, so that you may be careful to do according to all that is written in it. For then you will make your way prosperous, and then you will have good success (Joshua 1:8).

The only way to battle unproductive thoughts is with the Word of Truth. Joshua suggests meditating on it day and night. If that seems a bit overzealous, go to the questions above and remind yourself how often you fantasize about nutrient-less snacks. Overzealous?

Put on Prayer

"When we work, *we* work. When we pray, God works." Author unknown

E.M. Bounds was an American pastor, author, and lawyer who wrote a provocative little book published posthumously in 1958 entitled *Power through Prayer*. [Oliphants Ltd, London] He states, "The (Holy Ghost) does not anoint plans, but men – men of prayer." If we are earnest about God changing our idolatrous heart, we must put on prayer daily. Robert Murray McCheyne is quoted as saying, "Luther spent his best three hours in prayer."

George Muller was an 18th century pastor best known for his work building Christian homes and schools for orphans. Though the ministry slowly grew to house over 10,000 children, he never owed a penny. He believed God meant what He said in Romans 13:8, *owe no man anything.* His autobiography is inspiring (and a bit convicting . . .) as he describes his daily – sometimes hourly – dependence on God for food and supplies. Literally, day after day for years, just as their cupboards were bare, someone would bless them with a sovereign (an English gold coin), and sometimes multiple pounds. I have dog-eared several of his statements; here are a few of my favorites.

> "The greatness of the sum required to accomplish this work gives me special joy. The greater the difficulty to be overcome, the more it will be seen how much can be accomplished by prayer and faith. (5/24/1851)

> "The less that comes in, the more earnestly I pray, the more I look out for answers, and the more assured I am that the Lord, in His own time, will send me all I need." (6/21/1851)

> "How different, if one waits for God's own time and looks to Him for help and deliverance! When at last help comes, after many hours of prayer and after much faith and patience, how sweet it is!" (10/9/1853) [*The Autobiography of George Muller*, Whitaker House]

George Muller dramatically altered the lives of thousands of orphans, not because he was savvy or shrewd, but because he was a man of fervent prayer.

Intellectually most Christians would give an acknowledging nod to prayer. "Prayer moves the hand of God," we tout. But be honest, what does your prayer life look like? If God were your earthly partner, how intimate would you rate the relationship? How well do you know Him and how much of your life and heart have you shared with Him? Do you regularly sit and intentionally listen for His still small voice, or are you more prone to arrow prayers, a handful of sentences rocketed upward in moments of crisis? Richard Foster's book entitled *Prayer* states: "To believe that God can reach us and bless us in the ordinary junctures of daily life is the stuff of prayer." [*Prayer, Finding the Heart's True Home,* Harper Collins, p. 11]

Prayer requires quiet time alone, and we are called. We are called to pray about everything. Do you? If it's a regular routine, how do you feel when you miss it? If you're not consistent, what needs to happen to make that happen?

_____

_____

Do you have categories of challenges you bring to the Lord, and those you don't? Muse for a moment:

_____

_____

What keeps you from prayer time? Consider both internal and external obstacles.

_____

_____

Do you think your prayer life has any impact on your resolve to eat more healthfully and move more frequently? If so, how?

_____

_____

What is your next right step? To what would you like your friend or group to hold you accountable?

_____

_____

I've been consistent in my prayer time for a while, but my journey of turning definitely changed the content and tone. Historically, in addition to intercession for my unsaved friends and family, I diligently sought God's guidance. From major purchases to investing my time according to His will, my days began at my prayer desk. Unfortunately, that didn't change my stony heart.

Remember Paul Tripp's recommendation? "You already have a new heart. You have been radically changed by his grace and are being progressively restored day by day. The only way to properly celebrate these realities is to humbly ask, 'God, where are you calling me to further change? What qualities that you promise to your children are still not active in my heart? What do you want me to see about you?'" [_How People Change_, Paul Tripp, p. 117]

You reflected on Tripp's questions earlier, but let's do it again. Has anything changed?

God, where are you calling me to further change?

What qualities that you promise to your children are still not active in my heart?

What do you want me to see about you?

Though I continued to pray from the crumpled paper in my pocket, *I will sprinkle clean water on you, and you shall be clean from all your uncleannesses, and from all your idols I will cleanse you . . . ,* I added to my petitions. "Lord, what else? What idols other than anger do you want me to face?" As they say, be careful what you pray for. I'll share later.

We are called to cast our cares upon our Lord, but have you asked Him to help you with your physical discipline? Have you claimed His strength, or do you rely on your own willpower? Miss Grace offers her advice here: https://www.livewellbygrace.com/speaking-blog/2018/10/28/god-power-not-willpower

Consider each of the following verses relative to your resolve to elevate your commitment to self-care.

⁷Ask, and it will be given to you; seek, and you will find; knock, and it will be opened to you. ⁸For everyone who asks receives, and the one who seeks finds, and to the one who knocks it will be opened (Matthew 7:7-8).

If you don't already, how can you pray specifically regarding your body maintenance activities? i.e. Find an accountability buddy, learn simple food prep, support someone else?

_____

_____

When your brain is luring you toward derailment, how can you avail yourself of His steadfastness for your strength? His steadfastness for your strength?

_____

_____

How many times a day does your heart yearn for help? Whether it's with sustaining your fitness plan or holding your tongue (sometimes tougher than eating your greens . . .), it would be nice to have some hand holding. Ask and ye shall receive. His aid awaits. James 4:7-8 says, *Submit yourselves therefore to God. Resist the devil, and he will flee from you.* Don't you love that? Envision the devil running for his sorry life, dodging the

BEHOLD HIM | CHAPTER 8

power of Christ in you. *Draw near to God, and He will draw near to you.* Experience the strength of a spirit-filled snuggle.

⁶do not be anxious about anything, but in everything by prayer and supplication with thanksgiving let your requests be made known to God. ⁷And the peace of God, which surpasses all understanding, will guard your hearts and your minds in Christ Jesus (Philippians 4:6-7).

Are you anxious about your health and habits? What would you like to share with your Father? It's never too late.

_____

_____

²⁰But you, beloved, building yourselves up in your most holy faith and praying in the Holy Spirit, ²¹keep yourselves in the love of God, waiting for the mercy of our Lord Jesus Christ that leads to eternal life (Jude 20-21).

Another sermon in a sentence: *Keep yourselves in the love of God.* Go back to the last time you *did not do what you wanted, but did the very thing you hate* (Romans 7:15). Kudos to Paul for his candor . . . Were you keeping yourself in God's love? Debrief.

_____

_____

Take a quick break and listen to Luke Bryan's song, Pray About Everything. And while you're listening, stand up and dance! https://www.youtube.com/watch?v=NLs8FamXyOo

Need Insight?

The prophet Isaiah, centuries before Jesus' birth, referred to Him as Wonderful Counselor (Isaiah 9:6). Are there areas of your life are you truly confused about what to do? Pray. What concerns make your heart heavy? Tell your Father. Do you have requests and confessions you'd like to share with Him? He is anxiously awaiting the conversation. Consider James words of wisdom below as you continue your commitment to praying about your food and fitness.

⁵If any of you lacks wisdom, let him ask God, who gives generously to all without reproach, and it will be given him (James 1:5).

One of the common questions you might ask when starting (or restarting . . .) a fitness program is how you are going to make it happen. When will you find the time? Are you honestly ready to shop (grocery, not retail therapy) and cook? Can you make appetizing meals? Will your family and friends be supportive? If not, how should you respond? In what areas do you need wisdom?

_____

_____

_____

Let us then with confidence draw near to the throne of grace, that we may receive mercy and find grace to help in time of need (Hebrews 4:16).

Embrace God's grace. We are called to "draw near with confidence" to the throne of grace of our empathetic, merciful, heavenly high priest. About what do you lack confidence in coming before His throne?

_____

_____

_____

Phrase Prayers

Above I used the description, "sermon in a sentence." The Bible is riddled with them. There are also innumerable prayers in a phrase. Most of us need to spend more open-ended, listening-above-speaking, contrite heart time with God. But meditating on short phrases sears an idea in your soul.

Consider the Biblical phrases below. As you slowly, deliberately, prayerfully read them, is your spirit stirred?

You are my God.
Holy is Thy name.
Thy word is truth.
Thy will be done.
Hope in God.

We are called to pray without ceasing. Choosing a daily phrase prayer is a great way to sustain an on-going connection with your Good Shepherd. Hour-by-hour, throughout your day, prayerfully whisper the phrase. It will transform your heart.

Read through Psalm 63 and 119, noting any phrases that feel like a prayer to you. Begin keeping a phrase prayer list for future reference. Record your favorites here.

_____

_____

_____

Speed Dial

Are you amazed that the Lord God Almighty has invited you to cast all your cares on Him? My pastor used a familiar, aggravating experience to underscore our privilege of direct access to God:

"You're already frustrated because some situation is forcing you to call Customer Service. Immediately you have to listen to 15 options and figure out the correct category. You press the extension and you immediately hear, 'Thank you for calling Customer Service. Due to a high call volume you may experience a longer wait time.' Great. Then the elevator music begins. You know you've been holding awhile when you can hum along with the tune on perpetual loop. Finally someone answers, but his accent is so thick you can't understand what he's saying. What time is it over there anyway? But what you can hear clearly, 'That is not my department. Let me transfer you. One moment.' Then click, back to the music loop. Until you hear a dial tone. You've been disconnected."

Does your blood pressure rise just reading this?

With God, there's no waiting. No mishaps. When you need wise counsel – or supernatural strength – or just a little love – He's immediately available 24/7/365.

NOTE: Have you ever called on Him, began the conversation, then *you* hung up?

Put on Faith

Faith is the assurance of things hoped for, the conviction of things not seen . . . And without faith it is impossible to please Him, for he who comes to God must believe that He is, and that He is a rewarder of those who seek Him (Hebrews 11:1,6, NASB). Two profoundly powerful statements.

Faith is the assurance of things hoped for, the conviction of things not seen. The confidence, certainty, sureness of things to come. As I asked God to sprinkle me with clean water – to give me a softer heart – I had to ask myself, "Do I believe He will?" Do you envision and expect God to answer your prayers for heart transformation, prompting physical change? Can you say with enthusiasm you are becoming a new creation? Reflect here:

_____

_____

_____

But faith transcends simply trusting. *Believing before seeing* is an important piece of the puzzle, but true faith also requires knowledge and action. Do you trust God because you have come to know Who He Is, or is it simply fingers-crossed, I'm-in-a-bind-so-what-do-I-have-to-lose faith? Go back and read all the stories of the faith-full in Hebrews 11. Each one had an inviolable, experiential, transformative knowledge of God and His goodness. To know Him is to trust Him.

Then there's action; "preparing your field," illustrated momentarily. Imagine a little girl jumping from the top of the slide into her father's extended arms. She is absolutely certain of her dad's ability and trustworthiness in catching her, so she leaps with joyful abandon. Do you believe in God's goodness enough to bound into obedience behind Him? To know Him is to trust Him, and to trust Him is to follow Him.

And without faith it is impossible to please Him, . . . That definitely steps it up a notch. If I don't believe He can and He will, He will be displeased. "Trust Me, Judith. I *will* sprinkle clean water over you. I *will* give you a new heart. You can't change on your own. You know this because you've tried. How many times have you tried? Trust Me. I have begun a good work in you. I will do it."

Disbelief reveals doubt in God's ability, love, mercy, grace and faithfulness.

Lord, help me in my unbelief.

Do you believe?

for he who comes to God must believe that He is, . . .

Here's the truth that pushes me over the line. *He who comes to God must believe that He IS.*

"If the people of Israel ask me your name, what shall I say to them?" Moses asked God.

He replied, "I AM WHO I AM."

God said to Judith, "I AM WHO I AM."

Transformation isn't about you – it's about God, the great I AM.

Ponder that a moment and write your thoughts.

_____

_____

_____

. . . and that He is a rewarder of those who seek Him.

As the product of an earthly father who rarely rewarded, this was a tough concept for me, but there it was in black-and-white. He rewards what? My diligent efforts? No, He rewards those who *seek* Him – who read His Word and listen for His voice in earnest prayer.

Paul explicitly explains God's grace through faith in his letter to the Romans. Let's look at chapters 3 and 4.

Romans 3:9-20 No one is righteous through his own efforts

Romans 3:21-31 We are deemed righteous solely through faith in Jesus Christ

Romans 4 Abraham received the promise of becoming "father of many nations" through the righteousness of faith.

Romans 4:20-21 is worthy of printing, regular reading, and ultimately memorizing: [20]*No unbelief made him waver concerning the promise of God, but he grew strong in his faith as he gave glory to God,* [21]*fully convinced that God was able to do what he had promised.*

Do you sometimes doubt you'll ever be fully healed, then become fearful, depressed, irritable, or prone to emotional eating? It is important to recognize and give God glory for what He has and is doing in your life, even if you haven't yet seen the full revelation. Acknowledge and thank Him here for your small steps of success.

_____

_____

Are you *fully convinced His is able*? Read 2 Corinthians 9:8 for additional faith fueling: *God is able to make all grace abound to you, so that having all sufficiency in all things at all times, you may abound in every good work.*

_____

_____

Many are familiar with Proverbs 3:5-6: *Trust in the Lord with all your heart and lean not on your own understanding. In all your ways acknowledge Him and He will make your paths straight.*

I have mentioned that I previously prayed mainly for direction and comfort vs. inner sanctification. I wanted straight paths for maximum efficiency. 😊 But when I reflect back on my anger-instigated digressions, it's clear I still needed to look to Him for my heart change too. How about you? Where have you been leaning on your own understanding vs. trusting the Lord?

_____

_____

_____

Testimonials fuel faith. When we see other sisters tearing down strongholds, we begin to believe we can too. Take some time to read about Kimberly Taylor's journey, and for regular encouragement and inspiration, join her Take Back Your Temple program: http://www.TakeBackYourTemple.com

Here's what we know: God's Word is more powerful than any two-edged sword. You become a new creation through the renewing of your mind. We go back to Who God Is and what He has promised. "The only way you can wrestle yourself down is by the promises of God. You need help the way a drowning man needs help from outside himself to rescue him." [David Powlison, *Seeing With New Eyes*, p. 81]

Read and reflect on how the verses below can help you stay in faith in your fitness:

He who began a good work in you will perfect it until the day of Christ (Philippians 1:6).

I have been crucified with Christ. It is no longer I who live, but Christ who lives in me. And the life I now live in the flesh I live by faith in the Son of God, who loved me and gave himself for me (Galatians 2:20).

Writing a workbook is an arduous process. I definitely had some dips in faith along the way. "Why bother?" I asked myself. "No one will read it . . ." But believing God had given me the message and motivation, I plugged my ears to unbelief and contracted a talented young man to create my cover. Once I had that visual, how could I possibly punt?

Evidence of believing is envisioning. Planning. Remember, *faith is the assurance of things hoped for, the conviction of things not seen.* Have you ever fallen into discouragement because the scale's not moving? You've been walking and starving (it seems . . .) and nothing's happening. Those are Ys in the road. Will you continue in faith, or veer into the dessert ditch?

There is a compelling segment in the movie *Facing the Giants* where a story is told of two farmers, both of whom prayed for rain to rescue their fields from a long drought. Only one, though, went out and prepared his field to receive it. "Which one do you think trusted God to send the rain?"

Here's the clip: https://www.youtube.com/watch?v=WAxwS8KyMQQ&t=4s

What is your next step of active faith? What do you need to do to prepare your field?

_____

_____

Keep Luke 17:5-6 close at hand: *The apostles said to the Lord, "Increase our faith!" And the Lord said, "If you had faith like a grain of mustard seed, you could say to this mulberry tree, 'Be uprooted and planted in the sea,' and it would obey you.*

Galatians 2:20 is an arousing optic. *I have been crucified with Christ. It is no longer I who live, but Christ who lives in me. And the life I now live in the flesh I live by faith in the Son of God, who loved me and gave himself for me.*

How can this verse influence your health goals?

_____

_____

Let's face it, the journey is hard. It's like golf: good days and bad days. You have experienced the sweet joy of self-control through the Spirit, and the disappointment of failure. Like ABC's Wide World of Sports, you have known the _____ of victory and the _____ of defeat. C'mon old folks. Do you remember the 1970's ad? For the young'uns, here's a cheat:

https://www.youtube.com/watch?v=P2AZH4FeGsc

What do you do when you're crippled by doubt? Turn to the Word.

Fear not, for I am with you; be not dismayed, for I am your God; I will strengthen you, I will help you, I will uphold you with my righteous right hand (Isaiah 41:10).

Moment by moment, day after day, children of God must acknowledge their weakness and rely on the One Who is faithful. Regardless of the trial, large or small, we must rally our strength in the Spirit through His Word. Ingest it. Drink of the fount. Read it. Write it. Memorize it. Plaster it on the fridge. The only way to change your habits is to change your mind, and the only way to positively, permanently change your mind is to meditate on the Word!

Personalize and practice standing on the promises of God. Read this aloud, again and again and again. "I am not afraid, for my Father is with me. He will strengthen me. He will help me. He will uphold me with His righteous right hand."

Maybe it's not doubt or despair that's draggin' your wagon. Maybe you're just dog-tired. I mean, why wouldn't you be? Who works harder than women? You spend all day chasing the kids around, or are in a nutty office with nutty people, then fix supper while prodding the chillies to finish their homework. That is if you're not shuttling them off to some sport practice. And now you're supposed to add 30 minutes of walking? Yeah, right.

Though your schedule may be packed, your heart need not be burdened. Allow your Father to share the load. Hear His heart with this call: [28]*Come to me, all who labor and are heavy laden, and I will give you rest.*[29]*Take my yoke upon you, and learn from me, for I am gentle and lowly in heart, and you will find rest for your souls.*[30]*For my yoke is easy, and my burden is light* (Matthew 11:28-30).

Are there burdens are you needlessly carrying? How can you change your yoke?

_____

_____

One or more of the passages above surely strengthened your heart. Write them down. Read them regularly. Post them conspicuously. Memorize them. As John MacArthur says, "A Word-filled heart leaves no place for sin."

Speak the Truth

Reading God's word is transformational. Speaking it prompts power.

Read Psalm 46:1-3:

God is our refuge and strength, a very present help in trouble.
²Therefore we will not fear though the earth gives way,
    though the mountains be moved into the heart of the sea,
³though its waters roar and foam, though the mountains tremble at its swelling.

In what ways did this passage move you?

_____

_____

Envision someone in your family or small group is experiencing a trial. They have asked you to call on the Lord for strength. Stand up, take three deep breaths, and read the same passage aloud.

God is our refuge and strength, a very present help in trouble.
²Therefore we will not fear though the earth gives way,
    though the mountains be moved into the heart of the sea,
³though its waters roar and foam, though the mountains tremble at its swelling.

Did this audible proclamation impact you differently? How? Describe.

_____

_____

Sometimes circumstances demand powerful prose. Reading the Word softens the heart. Proclaiming the Word aloud strengthens the soul.

It Takes Two to Tango

Prayer and reading the Word are life-long partners. Like eating nutritiously and moving regularly, they are inseparable. Pastor John Piper says in his 12/30/01 sermon* "Prayer and meditation are inseparable, just like the Word and the Spirit are inseparable . . . God intends for your prayers to be saturated with Word, and the Word to be saturated with prayer . . . ."

---

* http://www.desiringgod.com; Hold Fast to the Word and Pray for Us, based on 2 Thessalonians 2:13-3:5

Do you personally pray scriptures? Turning the words into first person pleas? Praying through the Psalms is a great way to start, turning David's petitions into your own.

Lord, help me to delight in your law, meditating on it day and night (Psalm 1).

Father, instruct me and teach me in the way in which I should go. Guide me with Your eyes (Psalm 32:8).

I will extol you, My God and King, and bless your name forever and ever. Every day I will bless you and praise your name. Great are You, Lord, and greatly to be praised. Your greatness is unsearchable (Psalm 145:1-3).

And of course, Psalm 139 is full of personal prayers.

One of my favorites, especially in light of my belief that I have been called to stir up the church, is 2 Thessalonians 1:11-12. I pray it personally. "Lord, make me worthy of your calling. Fulfill my every resolve for good and every work of faith by Your power, so that Your name might be glorified."

Pastor Piper also recommends saturating God's Word with prayer. Before you begin your Bible reading, petition Him to open your heart, to block all distractions, that you would be transformed by His Spirit. Create in me a clean heart, O God, and renew a right spirit within me.

Saturate your prayers with the Word, and the Word with prayer.

Put on Praise

Praise befits the upright (Psalm 33:1).

We're called to praise God in worship. He wants all the glory. Sound a little Self-absorbed? Well . . . as He should be. God is very good to us and as Christ-followers we are blessed exceeding abundantly beyond belief, *and* God wants to be glorified in all we say and do. Let's look again at 2 Thessalonians 1:11-12: *To this end we always pray for you, that our God may make you worthy of his calling . . . so that the name of our Lord Jesus may be glorified in you, and you in him, according to the grace of our God and the Lord Jesus Christ.* All that we are, say, and do is to give God glory.

The Word clearly calls us to worship. To lift Him up. To acknowledge His goodness through praise. Read 1 Chronicles 16:23-36 and reflect on why we worship.

What is Worship?

How often do you worship? No, I didn't ask how frequently you attend church. I'd like you to consider how often you intentionally take time to honor and praise God. Only on Sundays? After He's given you a special, unexpected blessing? Throughout your days?

Worship isn't just singing on the Sabbath. It's actively honoring, uplifting, praising and thanking God. 1 Thessalonians 5:17 says *pray without ceasing.*

When you listen to the morning birdsong, do you thank God you can hear? _____

When you sit down to dine, are you grateful for the feast? _____

When you really don't feel like exercising, are you full of awe you are able? _____

"In everything, give thanks," says 1 Thessalonians 5:18. But I'm sure that excludes your food and fitness issues, right? Wrong. In everything, including your struggle to stay on track with your temple care, give thanks.

David Platt wisely says, "Worship isn't a spectator sport." In a sermon given when he was still at The Church at Brook Hills in Birmingham, AL, he identified three components to God-centered worship, 1. Revere His Greatness, 2. Relish His Presence, and 3. Reflect His Holiness. [Radical.net; God-centered worship, Mark 11:15-19, 4/9/06] We're going to look at each from a *physical* point of view.

Revere His Greatness

When was the last time you star gazed? On your next cloudless night, read Isaiah 40:25-26, then go out and praise God for His awesome creation.

Some will accuse, "Your God is too small." How about yours? You say He can do anything, but does that include changing your heart from abhorrence for exercise to enthusiasm? Can He tame your temptation to eat late at night? Is He bigger than that brownie? Reflect.

_____

_____

What if you considered physical self-care as an act of worship? Eating well would become a celebration. Exercising would be transformed into worship workouts™. Write some words, phrases, songs, and/or thoughts about how you can give God glory through your food and movement habits.

_____

_____

Look at the list of fruits and vegetables in Appendix 1. Have you gratefully received (aka: eaten) *all* God's bounty? Which ones have you obstinately overlooked? "I hate Brussels sprouts!" Could it be 'cus you steam them into mush? Would you consider a new-food-per-week plan, sharing your luscious concoctions with your church? Taste and see that the Lord is good!

Good health is a gift. To be able to go for a walk, feel your internal temperature climbing, your muscles moving, your breaths quickening and deepening is a gracious, divine gift. Consider how it feels to be sick, injured or otherwise bedridden. Tell your Father how much you appreciate your ability to get up and go.

Then go for a walk. Look up *Holy, Holy, Holy is the Lord* on YouTube and listen to your favorite rendition. While singing "the whole earth is full of His glory," notice the birds darting, flowers parading, and the generous gift of (wo)man's best friend.

Relish His Presence

Time and again through His Word, God promises never to leave nor forsake us. Isaiah 43:1-3 says *Fear not, for I have redeemed you; I have called you by name, you are mine. When you pass through the waters, I will be with you; and through the rivers, they shall not overwhelm you; when you walk through fire you shall not be burned, and the flame shall not consume you. For I am the Lord your God, the Holy One of Israel, your Savior.*

Then there's Deuteronomy 31:8, *The Lord, Himself, goes before you and will be there with you. He will never leave you nor forsake you. Do not be afraid; do not be discouraged.*

Pastor Platt says about relishing God's presence, "It's the most acknowledged truth but the least experienced promise of God."

Do you daily experience God's presence in your life? Do you actively listen for the Good Shepherd's voice?

_____

_____

When and where do you thank Him for being close by?

_____

_____

Do you speak to Him throughout your days like He's sitting shotgun? How can you elevate the conversation?

_____

When you are having a sugar craving, do you ask Him for help? Do some dittling here: (Don't you love this new word?)

_____

_____

If you honestly have difficulty feeling God's presence, ask Him to speak louder. Pray He make you aware of His love and attendance to you. Be specific about situations or circumstances when you need to know He's near. He'll be thrilled you asked . . .

Let's go back to Worship Workouts™. Do you pray when you walk? Use your Bluetooth and pretend you're talkin' to your bestie. (Well, you are.) What a great time to itemize all the things, large and small, you're grateful for, and to pray for those who are unable to enjoy being outside. What about singing while walking? Or dancing? Remember the prod, "Dance like no one's watching . . ." I dare ya.

Reflect His Holiness

God calls us to be holy. _Be ye holy as I am holy_ (1 Peter 1:16). That sure seems like a long shot, doesn't it? But as we discussed in Chapter 4, God already sees us as holy. If He weren't the awesome, all-knowing Maker you'd be tempted to question His judgment.

Holy means set apart; unique; different from the world. In his unsettling book, *Respectable Sins,* Jerry Bridges uses the example of the Air Force Academy to explain the idea of being set apart. He observes how different a cadet's experience is from the normal college kid. He writes,

> "Why is there this difference between the Academy and a typical university? These young men and women have been in a real sense 'set apart' by the U.S. government to become Air Force officers . . . .So the Academy doesn't exist to prepare young people to be schoolteachers or Wall Street bankers. It exists for one purpose: to prepare officers for the U.S. Air Force. And the cadets are 'set apart' for that purpose . . . .
>
> When I was serving as an officer in the U.S. Navy some fifty years ago, there was an expression: 'conduct unbecoming an officer.' That expression covered anything from minor offenses resulting in a reprimand to major ones requiring a court martial. But the expression was more than a description of aberrant behavior; it was a statement that the conduct was inconsistent with that expected of a military officer . . . .Perhaps we might do well to adopt a similar expression for believers: 'conduct unbecoming a saint.'" [*Respectable Sins,* NavPress, pp. 11-13]

As Christians, what does it mean to be set apart in the physical realm? As Americans are getting larger and larger, seems we are no different from the world. When foods are offered that have been unequivocally determined to undermine our health, do we choose differently? Going back to Relishing God's Presence, if you considered Him dining with you at every meal (He is, you know), would you change your menu?

Let me again be clear: I am *not* calling any foods sinful. (Well, maybe fried pork rinds are Satan's snack.) I'm simply suggesting a different perspective on creating new habits. If you believe God is calling you to better care for your health, because He cares for you, because He wants you to be set apart and live victoriously both spiritually and physically, then choosing cauliflower and hummus over Hot Pockets makes you holy! (You may need to sit with that one a minute . . .)

I desire steadfast love and not sacrifice, the knowledge of God rather than burnt offerings (Hosea 6:6).

David Platt's interpretation of that verse: "God is not honored by our religion; He is honored with our hearts and our obedience."

Consider this verse relative to your previous attempts at dieting. Think again about caring for your temple as an act of worship. Is this a paradigm shift for you? Note how you would describe to a friend your new way of thinking.

_____

_____

Let's Worship!

Ponder this formula: worship + thanksgiving = strength

Have you ever noticed that?

You're feeling down-in-the dumps. Unmotivated. The blues are nudging you to bail on your walk. What's a wobbler to do? Bring out the Book. Use the verses below in the coming weeks to lift up your voice to the Lord. Print them out and stick them in your pocket so you have a cheat sheet when you're walking and praising.

Nehemiah 9:5-6
Psalm 9:1-2
Psalm 66:1-4
Psalm 100

But don't stop there! Sing to the Lord a new (or old) song. _Tell of His deeds in songs of joy!_ (Psalm 107:22) Can you still remember your camp favorites from decades gone by? If not, just like your scriptures, print out inspiring song lyrics and pocket them. Here are a few guaranteed to move your heart and your hips. I dare you to stand up and sing along with Danniebelle below and stay down in the dumps.

O Se Baba https://www.youtube.com/watch?v=AGJGhVqNmw4

Garment of Praise https://www.youtube.com/watch?v=_ecb5Vu3N0Y

Remember this late great? WAIT for it! https://www.youtube.com/watch?v=VPpd-6X3tEo

Have you ever gotten the evil eye for being overly zealous in church? Oh, go for it. Be zealous. The church could use some shakin'.

My friend Grace has a few ideas about merging your worship and your walks. Listen to her podcast called Preppy Praise Walks. https://www.livewellbygrace.com/speaking-blog/2018/10/16/peppy-praise-walks

Put on People

We've been considering how to get better acquainted with God. The previous disciplines may seem worthy of your time and attention – prayer, reading God's Word, being intentional about worship and giving thanks. But connecting with Christians, well . . . not so much. We all have great excuses for missing church and bailing on Bible study. It's inconvenient. Boring. And the age-old "they're just a bunch of hypocrites." Yep, all have sinned and fall short of the glory of God. You'll fit right in.

I've always struggled with regularly attending church, sometimes more than others.

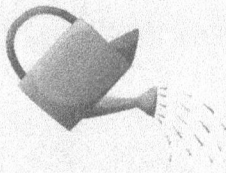

Judi's Journal 7/10/11

Out of guilt – sheer guilt – not joy or enthusiasm – this morning I went to church. And I'm riddled with angst. I DON'T want to be there! I don't want to sit through their crappy music – I simply don't want to do group worship. Or honestly, group anything.

Is that really so horrible a sin? What's wrong with wanting to do life – dinners, gatherings, worship – in smaller groups?

I was sitting there – ultimately crying – thinking "call me to shovel someone's porch – feed someone whos' sick – encourage a sister – but don't make me do group church!

Wow. That's some people-phobia right there. Why the aversion to church? What's behind the ranting?

I remember eating breakfast at a friend's house, and she asked me why my chair was so far from the table. I considered, then tears and sniffles surfaced. I knew it was irrational, but I admitted, "I need to be ready to run." Like the flight attendant's lecture before take-off, I always wanted to know where my exits were.

When Dad was home, dinners weren't pleasant. My mission was to get it finished so I could get out of the line of fire. When asked about school and homework, I knew if I didn't have a perfect report I'd have hell to pay, so suppers reinforced my belief that I am only safe alone.

Consider sitting in a sanctuary full of humans. I feel like cat caught in a corner with a pit bull baring its teeth. OK, maybe a bit exaggerated, but I do have an aversion to crowds and tight seating. (Airplanes?) I'm happy to stand in the back.

But . . . Church is part of God's communication with us. The first church described in Acts 2 *were together and had all things in common. And they were selling their possessions and belongings and distributing the proceeds to all, as any had need. And day by day, attending the temple together and breaking bread in their homes, they received their food with glad and generous hearts praising God and having favor with all the people. And the Lord added to their number day by day those who were being saved* (Acts 2:42-47). And we fuss about a weekly, 2-hour small group gathering?

Though daily devotions are critical to spiritual maturity, it's life's application that cements God's truths in our souls. It's easy to memorize Isaiah 41:10, but God's presence, help, and strength is oftentimes revealed through the Body of Christ. "The hands and feet of Jesus." Though the idea of gathering with the saints usually brings spiritual education and edification to mind, we all know a lot happens behind the scenes. Some churches embrace the phrase "Doing life together." Flowers at weddings. Casseroles at funerals. Seasonal celebrations. So why are we not doing temple-care together? After the personality tests are tallied, it's clear we all have different tastes, temperaments and talents, but everyone wants to be healthy. When we stir one another up spiritually, shall we not also exhort each other to physical earnestness? As stated in the introduction, the Church is highly committed to supporting one another in our spiritual and emotional growth, but talking about health (or lack of it) is taboo. Why? The Bible is rife with scriptures on strength by banning together as the Body of Christ.

Read 1 Corinthians 12:12-27.

If there are members in your church with a physical condition (hypertension, diabetes, heart disease), who must be diligent about altering their food and increasing their activity, how does that impact the entire church body? Are there ways to support them in these difficult lifestyle changes?

_____

_____

_____

9Two are better than one, because they have a good reward for their toil. 10For if they fall, one will lift up his fellow. But woe to him who is alone when he falls and has not another to lift him up! 11Again, if two lie together, they keep warm, but how can one keep warm alone? 12And though a man might prevail against one who is alone, two will withstand him—a threefold cord is not quickly broken (Ecclesiastes 4:9-12).

Have you ever tried to diet or undertake a new exercise regimen by yourself? How did that work out?

_____

_____

_____

Does your involvement in a body of believers impact your commitment to care for your health positively, negatively, or not at all?

_____

_____

_____

Is a buffet of sweets at church functions difficult for you when you're "trying to be good"?

_____

_____

_____

Dr. Paul Tripp comments about the church and change: "Our fellowship is an essential ingredient for lasting change . . . change is something God intends his people to experience together. It's a corporate goal. What God does in individuals is part of a larger story of redemption that involves all of God's people." [Paul Tripp, *How People Change*, pp. 65-66]

Jesus said, *"He who is not for me is against me."* (Matthew 12:30) Unfortunately, this also holds true in your earthly relationships, even within the Church. There are people who uplift and encourage, and there are those who pull you down. There are those who honor and support your commitment to personal self-care, while others scoff and sabotage. One of the best ways to strengthen your own commitment and resolve is to encourage others. I wholeheartedly believe the best way to stay on track is to support someone else . . . though a brownie might prevail against one who is alone, two will withstand him—a threefold cord is not quickly broken. 😊

Who in your church and/or community would be blessed by you uplifting them in their food and fitness? How do the verses below encourage sisterly support?

_____

_____

_____

24And let us consider how to stir up one another to love and good works, 25not neglecting to meet together, as is the habit of some, but encouraging one another, and all the more as you see the Day drawing near (Hebrews 10:24-25).

16Let the word of Christ dwell in you richly, teaching and admonishing one another in all wisdom, singing psalms and hymns and spiritual songs, with thankfulness in your hearts to God (Colossians 3:16).

Take a moment to think of the people in your church community who want to establish healthy habits. How can you help them? Will that motivate you too?

_____

_____

_____

Miss Grace has some thoughts:
https://www.livewellbygrace.com/speaking-blog/2019/9/23/help

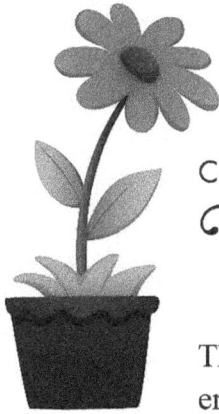

CHAPTER 9

Unbundle Your Stumble

The road to sanctification is hilly, rife with peaks and valleys. Having engaged in The Lab experiments, you now find yourself regularly eating breakfast, enjoying more fruits and vegetables than you previously knew existed, and are actually looking forward to your evening walks. Then you host your kid's 8th birthday party . . . Next, we'll spotlight a few of the most common sources of stumbling.

I slowly began to tepidly believe that I could, by God's grace, become a calm and kind new creation. Judi and gentle could be sheepishly muttered in the same sentence. But like most things for me, it wasn't happening fast enough for my liking. (Old idols die hard.) After such diligent repentance and prayer, like so many of those Jesus touched, I thought I'd be instantly, completely healed. My anger would forever be in my rearview mirror. Past tense.

Not so.

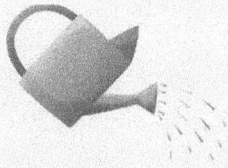

Lowes

When I received the email late Friday afternoon that my dishwasher had arrived at my local Lowes, I was surprised to read, "For your protection, only the cardholder or an authorized user of the credit card may pick up this purchase." Anxious to wrap up my work day and get Boaz out for a walk, I logged into my account to add my friend's name who would be picking it up for me. Much to my chagrin, there was no link to Add a New Card Holder. So, 1-800 was my only option.

Of course, the first step is always navigating the automated system. After entering my Lowes credit card number and password, it couldn't verify me. After three tries, I called again, was forced to listen to three rounds of extension options before finally I could press 0 to speak to a live person.

When the young woman came on the line asking for my account number, I immediately let her know I'd been greatly inconvenienced.

"I shouldn't even have to talk to you. I'm simply trying to add someone to my credit card. There was no way to do it online, which forces me to waste both my time and yours."

"I apologize for your frustration, ma'am. Before I can help you, I will need to verify your account. Can you please give me the last four digits of your social security number?"

"5-2-3-6."

"And what is the address on the account?"

Address provided.

"What was the amount of your last payment?"

"Are you kidding me? You're treating me like a convict, not a customer! How many questions do I need to answer before I can spend money at your store?" My computer was sitting nearby, so I located the last statement and gave her the information she requested. "Now can I add my friend to my account? The dishwasher needs to be picked up tomorrow."

"I just have a few more questions to verify your account."

"Are you serious? I'm not buying a house; I'm just trying to add someone to my credit card! Do you harass all your customers this way?"

"I apologize, ma'am. I'm just following protocol. Can you please give me the phone number associated with this account?"

I curtly, slowly, distinctly, semi-shouted the ten digits.

Finally, she verified my account, but said, "I'm sorry, but I can't help you add another authorized user."

"Are you flipping kidding me?! Why in the world are you making this so difficult? I'm trying to pick up a dishwasher I bought from you and I'm being interrogated like a felon. I need to speak with your supervisor."

"One moment please."

More waiting . . .

"Hello, this is Mrs. Graham. How can I help you?"

"All I'm trying to do is add someone to my credit card account. I tried to do it online and that wasn't possible. Your IT people should be fired. Then after being ridiculously questioned by your colleague she tells me she can't add another authorized user. This is outrageous. Can you P-L-E-A-S-E add my friend to the account?"

"I'm sorry, but you'll need to submit the information in writing."

"This is ridiculous. The dishwasher is already in. He wants to pick it up tomorrow. Can I email you the information?"

"No, I don't have access to email, but you can fax it."

"Fax it. Right. Who has a fax these days? You might mention to Lowes that this is the 21st century. I swear I'm cancelling this account and will never shop here again."

"I'm sorry ma'am. Have you tried to eFax? Let me give you the number."

I took down the number, said "Thank you for nothing," and hung up.

I felt like I was going to wretch. I was imprisoned by incompetence. I would have cancelled the order but I had already ordered from Appliance Connection who promised it by July 3rd, so when I called on July 6th (of course, the tracking link didn't work . . .), they said there had been a two-week delay. "Could you have notified me? Cancel the order." So, I had to get this stupid "written authorization" to these bimbos.

After twenty minutes of searching eFax apps for Android, installing and uninstalling four different ones that required me to pay for "credits", as a last resort, (I know, don't say it. I could have paid for the dang credits), I called the local store.

"Lowes Customer Service."

"I hope you can help me. I have a dishwasher there waiting for pick-up . . ."

She interrupted me. "What is the name on the account?"

I gave her my name.

"Yes, it arrived three days ago."

Not a surprise I received the email three days late . . .

"I only received the email notice today, which explicitly states whoever picks up the dishwasher must be an authorized user on my credit card."

"You can have anyone you want pick it up. We don't care. I just need to add his name to your order."

"Seriously? I just spent an hour going around and around and around with your online people because their notice clearly states my friend's name needs to be on my credit card."

"If you give me his name, I'll make a note and he can pick it up any time."

"R-O-N-B-R-A-N-T"

"Ron Brant. Perfect. He's noted on your order. Can I help you with anything else?"

"Yes, you can have your supervisor call me. The nightmare I just endured only hurts *you*, the stores. Lowes IT is clearly incompetent. It notified me three days late, told me Ron had to be listed as an authorized user of my card, trying to add him was a quagmire, and it was all a waste of time."

"But he can pick up the dishwasher any time, no problem!" She was trying to be chipper. "Can I help you with anything else?"

I was airing my grievances in vain. She didn't care. She had other customers waiting and wanted to get this crazy lady off the phone.

"No. Thanks for your help. Good-bye."

I was frazzled.

Predictably, I was wide awake at 3 a.m. feeling frustrated, not with Lowes but with myself. It happened again. I blew up because *I* had been inconvenienced. Yes, their system is convoluted and broken, but the women were just doing their jobs. I was nauseated with remorse. I stumbled from a relaxing, enjoyable Friday evening into angst and anger. I was back in bondage.

In this life there will be missteps.

We now understand we all have idols that lure us toward temptation. I covet my comfort and yell at people; you turn to food. Neither of us, in that moment, are walking in the Spirit. Jeremiah 17:9 reads *the heart is deceitful above all things, and desperately sick; who can understand it?* Overriding that sick heart requires a day-by-day, moment-by-moment, dying to me and seeking the Spirit. Period. There are also predictable potholes to be acknowledged and avoided. Let's consider some sources of stumbling.

Busyness/Time

Boy are we busy. And that's good, right? We're doing good deeds and accomplishing important things. But are you too busy to care for the Holy Spirit's house? Let's be honest: Satan *loves* an over-booked saint. He's dancing when you're stretched thin and exhausted, too busy to tend to your temple. What does the Word say about busy? Read the Martha/Mary story in Luke 10:38-42. You'd think being the hostess with the mostest would get Martha a kudo call-out but instead, Jesus suggested she sit a spell. Which are you? Mary or Martha? Is it impacting your take-care-of-you time?

Watch this video: https://vimeo.com/105381209

Sit and assess: To what am I giving time that is less important than weekly grocery shopping/food prep and regular exercise?

_____

_____

_____

My busy is a fantasy. Many of my bouts with anger and/or frustration stem from me thinking I don't have time for this, when in fact, my afternoon schedule could be clear. Whether it's a traffic jam or a slow grocery line (How many coupons does that lady have?), my prideful ego is incensed that the task has exceeded my self-determined timetable.

Comfort

Everyone craves comfort. Few purposely stand in the rain, live in a cold house, or stay up late working. We all prefer to be safely tucked into our cozy cocoon watching the Hallmark channel.

Oftentimes when asked about what motivates a person to choose certain unhealthy foods, they glibly respond, "Because it tastes good!" (Bless you, Aunt Helen.) Can you hear your inner self saying that? Now, in a sane moment, how is that strategy working for you? Cite specific examples.

_____

_____

_____

_____

Comfort is my idol. Having never been married, I have spent my entire adult life doing as I please, when I please, with whom (or not) I please. As I have mentioned, my peaceful serenity became my functional god. I wasn't happy if anyone disrupted my bliss.

There are foods that can create a feeling of comfort, mostly nutrient-void. I've never heard anyone say, "I was feeling sad so I ate a plate of sautéed asparagus." Do you turn to certain foods when you are in need of solace? Is this a pothole worth pondering? Capture the Holy Spirit's nudge (before you forget . . .):

_____

_____

_____

_____

Convenience

Have you ever yelled at someone because they happened to be the unfortunate person in your path? The flag person holding up your lane? A customer service rep? Your kids or spouse? Few of the victims of my rage are people I know. They are nameless and faceless. They are simply the poor sap who got the unlucky number to take my call or service my line.

When was the last time you mindlessly inhaled something unhelpful because . . . it was there. The M&Ms at your colleague's desk. The chips immediately served at your favorite Mexican restaurant. The pumpkin bread at Sunday School. (Pumpkin is healthy, right?) Then there's the convenience of the drive-thru. Just like the candy bars that call out your name at the check-out counter, spontaneous indulgences are rarely nutrient rich. What scripture and strategy can you institute to combat the enticement of convenience?

Social

We influence each other. We all make decisions affected by the opinions and lifestyle of those around us. Do you remember when it was total taboo to wear white socks, and wide belts and hip huggers were all the rage? And let's not kid ourselves, those closest to us can be the most unrelenting. Ever have Aunt Evelyn insist you eat her German chocolate cake she made especially for you? Fortunately, Aunt E's cake is an infrequent occurrence, but what about your close friendships? Do those relationships positively or negatively impact your food and fitness choices? Do your social activities revolve around food, or activity? Take a moment to consider how your behavior is impacted by your inner circle. If there's room for improvement, note ideas for positive change.

It's easy to overindulge with food. It's how we celebrate and socialize. As we relax with our tribe, it's tempting to amplify the comfortable connecting with unrestrained and unhealthy eating. Describe the satisfaction you feel when dining without restrictions. Why does it feel nurturing?

Next, reflect on a time you completely let down, had fun, and over ate. How did you feel afterwards? What things did you say to yourself later? Use as many descriptive words as are applicable.

_____

_____

One might ask, if it's not a big deal, why do we feel guilty afterwards?

According to your own reflections, can your food choices negatively impact your emotions and self-image? Explain:

_____

_____

How do your food choices impact others?

_____

_____

Does your call to love others and not make them stumble (1 Corinthians 8:7-12) impact your thinking when dining with friends and family? If so, how so? If not, why not?

_____

_____

Above I said: "As we relax with our tribe it's tempting to amplify the comfortable connecting with unrestrained and unhealthy eating." Socializing is a critical component for an abundant life. We need to bond with brothers and sisters, and we always want to give thanks to the Lord for His bountiful provision of food. The obvious question is, can we enjoy the fellowship of the saints without sabotaging ourselves? Consider the foods, especially sweets of all kinds, that are unfailingly found at church gatherings. What substitutes would be satisfying, but not sabotaging?

_____

_____

What strategies can you establish (ideally in cahoots with a buddy) to avoid unwise choices at group gatherings?

_____

_____

There is some (not enough . . .) debate, especially as it relates to the sacred cow of desserts, about regularly offering sweets after church considering at least 30% of the congregation has a physician's mandate to limit sugar consumption. Can we better love our neighbor by not tempting them with harmful foods? Honestly ponder.

Then there's the intrusive social media. How many food photos do you view every day? Can you remember a recent time when you were prompted by someone's post to eat something unwholesome? If you are active on-line, consider how declaring your 10:31 Habits (found in The Lab) and encouraging others to join you could strengthen your dedication, and theirs.

Clamor for Control

Self-control is a misnomer. As we've been discussing, we aspire to Spirit-control, stifling self-control. But since the final fruit mentioned in Galatians 5:22 is self-control, who are we to rephrase?

Let's start by asking, why might God call us to self-control? Let's go back to Ephesians 4:22-24: [20]*But that is not the way you learned Christ!—* [21]*assuming that you have heard about him and were taught in him, as the truth is in Jesus,* [22]*to put off your old self, which belongs to your former manner of life and is corrupt through deceitful desires,* [23]*and to be renewed in the spirit of your minds,* [24]*and to put on the new self, created after the likeness of God in true righteousness and holiness.*

God wants us to be new. Renewed. Done with the old destructive desires and behaviors. He wants my caustic spirit gone, and your lethargic, achy body behind you. That requires self-control, managing your brat.

Spend any time with young children and it becomes clear that brattiness is inbred. We all have that inner, selfish kid demanding our way. That petulant child is in direct conflict with the Spirit, who wants us to surrender to His way. Our clamor for control was passed down from Adam and Eve, but as we daily die to self, the Holy Spirit overcomes our feisty flesh.

Tricia used to say, "A slip-up isn't a relapse." My phraseology is, we stumble our way to sanctification. You *will* fail, but by God's grace you will get up and begin walking again.

Examine situations and/or times of day when your inner brat gets raucous. Note specific strategies for stifling her by the Spirit.

_____

_____

_____

Anti-Tripping Tips

As stated earlier, "The road to sanctification is hilly, rife with peaks and valleys." There is absolutely no better system for tempering our tripping than the power of prayer, reading God's Word, praising Him and communing with His people. But, you do have some other strategic tools in your toolbox that will minimize slips and falls.

Be a Buddy

A good friend is a beacon and a buoy. She directs you toward the Light, uplifts you when you're wavering, and stirs you to fuel well and move often. The best thing about buddies is the reciprocity; be a buddy, get a buddy. Following are some Buddy Basics.

1. **Bible-based** Though you want to nurture non-Christian friendships, only those who speak the Word into your life can positively impact your transformation process. The same holds true when encouraging your friends. Read passages like Hebrews 12:1-17 together, *considering Him who endured from sinners such hostility against Himself, so that you may not grow weary or fainthearted* (Hebrews 12:3).
2. **Loyal** I'll never forget the dreadful day my Rhodesian Ridgeback, in the prime of his life, ate a poison mushroom and I found myself at the emergency vet, sobbing hysterically to my friend. Though I was 90 miles away, she arrived in less than two hours. *A friend loves at all times, and a brother is born for adversity* (Proverbs 17:17). Friends are there for you, come rain or shine. They walk with you in good times and bad, messy and momentous.
3. **Grace-Full** Friends are fallible. Expect disappointment. Life happens. But forgiveness heals the wound and strengthens the bond. As mirrors of God's love, friends are full of grace, abounding in steadfast love.
4. **Balanced** Have you ever had a "friend" who would call and immediately release an avalanche of blather? You could put down the phone, go do your dishes, and

come back later and she'd still be rambling? Then ironically, when she finally stops to take a breath, she says, "Great to talk to you," and hangs up. She ain't no friend. Conversation can be a telling test of the relational symmetry. Good pals both give and receive.

5. **Honest** Candor counts. A real friend will warn you – even exhort you – when you are heading down a perilous path. And if you persist and tumble down the precipice, she's there to hoist you out. Take note: Be picky. If you are entangled with someone who's incessantly stumbling, despite your encouragement, prayers, and intervention in her life, it may be time to reassess their prominence in yours.

Be picky when picking your pals. We all have vulnerable times and circumstances when we may be prone to join the wrong pack. We want to be seen in that circle. We enjoy the activity. We're just plain lonely and would hang out with anyone who would welcome us. Proverbs 18:24 prods us to be particular. *A man of many companions may come to ruin, but there is a friend who sticks closer than a brother.* Like the Bible's warning about wolves, the wrong friends can lure you down dangerous paths. Listen to a lesson by Grace: https://www.livewellbygrace.com/speaking-blog/2018/10/28/broken-yokes

Ask for Accountability

While you share the inner sanctum of your heart with your close friends, accountability buddies can be anyone. You are merely looking for folks to hold you to your new habits, and vice versa. That can be your pickleball pals, bunko buddies, and/or friends far away. In fact, the more accountability you have, the more guardrails to keep you from skidding off the road.

Establish a Specific Schedule

Plan your work and work your plan. A variety of commitments crowd your calendar. Work. Kid's activities. Church. What days and times will you walk? Is that also when you'll stretch a bit and sprinkle in some strength training? I once knew a gal who kept her fitness ball in the basement, and did two minutes of abs every time she downed the stairs. If you leave it to chance – when you have time – it won't happen. Meal prep requires the same commitment. When will you grocery shop, and what block in your calendar is for cooking? Make some notes:

To assist with your consistent assessment, Exhibit 5 offers you a Weekly Reckoning, which is simply a template for asking yourself how you're doing. For full effect, share your answers with your buddy.

Target Compelling Achievements

Which sounds more stirring, I want to lose ten pounds, or I want to comfortably complete the Wag & Walk fundraiser for the local humane society? Would you prefer to go on a diet, or to try new vegetarian recipes? Will you take a sculpting class because you should, or to support your friend who invited you to join her? It seems obvious, but how many people still attempt to alter their deeply-entrenched routines for the gloomy goal of losing a few pounds? List three ways you can make your fitness journey meaningful. Significant. Rewarding. Purpose-full.

1. _____

2. _____

3. _____

Beware of Boredom

Boredom begets bailing. Like all things in life, it's important to stir up your food and fitness lest it grow stale. Are you unenthused with your menu? Try a new recipe. Does everything taste bland? Go to Trader Joes and find an exotic sauce and/or salsa. When was the last time you added capers or sprinkled saffron? Exercise can become tedious too. Find a new route. Drive to a park or other pretty place. Are you adding exercises along the way, like push-ups off a felled tree, or crunches in a green meadow? A few pages back you listed three specific ways you would make your exercise fun. Have you implemented those great ideas? Given they are hereafter deemed Worship Workouts™, how could communing with your Creator ever become tiresome?

Tracking

According to Kaiser Permanente, keeping a food journal can double your weight loss. (https://about.kaiserpermanente.org/our-story/health-research/news/keeping-a-food-diary-doubles-diet-weight-loss-kaiser-permanente-) Do you really want to see Snickers candy bar permanently printed on a page? Let's look at some other statistics worth tracking.

Recording your fat grams can be enlightening, but remember all fats aren't created equal. Though we shunned all fats in decades past, unsaturated fats have been officially welcomed back into the grocery cart because they're full of valuable nutrients.

Watch this video: https://vimeo.com/125808853

But remember if you're attempting to lose weight, *all* fats are 9 calories per gram, compared to only 4 in carbs and proteins. So, if you're trying to reel in your calories, eat fats judiciously, keeping total daily intake under 50 grams.

Watch this video: https://vimeo.com/38373698

We discussed the detrimental effects of sugar, so let's start logging. Do you normally note the number of grams in everything you eat, limiting your daily consumption?

Watch this video: https://vimeo.com/38377131

Add a sugar column in your journal, topping your tally at 30-50 grams per day.

Tracking doesn't always need to carry an undercurrent of fear and shame. Sure, noting sugar and fat helps to corral the cravings, but it's surely more fun to watch the foods for which you get gold stars. We've already mentioned that fruits and veggies are a nutritional boon, so give yourself credit for consuming. What if you vowed to eat one or more food of every color every day? The rainbow diet!

Watch this video: https://vimeo.com/45814261

And remember we mentioned targeting 25 grams of fiber each day? Track it!

Tracking: Paper or Public?

Ready to start logging your life? There's an app for that! Track everything that slides between your teeth. Most have a huge database of foods, including popular brands. Some even allow you to enter your own creative concoctions. We didn't discuss logging your exercise earlier (didn't want to overwhelm you), but most apps include that too. Some even monitor your heart rate. (If only they'd come cook for you...) If you're a social sort, you can invite your friends to provide a friendly prod, and give each other a high five when you accomplish self-set goals. A few of the most popular are MyFitnessPal, LoseIt, Fooducate, Strava, MapMyFitness, ... I know, I've overlooked your favorite. Sorry.

Have you ever tracked your food before? Was that a positive experience? If so, why did you quit? Reflect back on what you learned.

_____

_____

Celebrate Success

Have you ever set an outlandish goal? A grand accomplishment within a short time period? It happens invariably in January. Though he hasn't had on a pair of running shoes in over a decade, he's going to lose 25 pounds and run the LA marathon come summer. Could that, in part, be why he's disillusioned by Valentine's Day?

We sabotage ourselves with overzealousness. Small steps make a *big* difference. What if your goal was to eat a healthy breakfast six out of seven days every week for the next three months? Not so exciting? It will be after you've dropped superfluous pounds.

Small, attainable goals, measured often and celebrated meaningfully is the formula for success. And remember, your focus is health & fitness, *not* weight loss. Given the overriding mandate to eat real food, and The Big 10 presented in The Lab, what small steps will you set for yourself, and how will you celebrate? (No ice cream sundaes, please.)

_____

_____

_____

_____

_____

_____

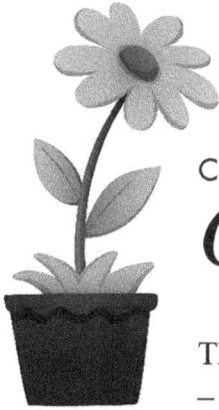

CHAPTER 10
Our Pleas, His Power

The Word is filled with God's promises to walk with us – to strengthen us – to be our ever-present help in trouble. This includes times of temptation. Our petitions for assistance are a sweet fragrance to our Father. What if you prayed the following verses, seeking self-control and resolve. Write each in first person personal tense. (Don't think that's an accepted grammatical phrase, but I like it.) i.e. Lord, You will command . . .

He will command His angels concerning you, to guard you in all your ways (Psalm 91:11).

The eyes of the Lord are on the righteous and His ears are open to their prayer (1 Peter 3:12).

The Lord is good, a stronghold in the day of trouble. He knows those who take refuge in Him (Nahum 1:7).

Each of these is a confession of faith. Print them out, keep them in your pocket, and speak them aloud often.

. . . for His glory.

We are made in the image of God (Gen 1:26), slowly becoming more like Christ (Romans 8:29), called to be holy and blameless (Col 1:20-23, Eph 1:4), all for *His* glory. Your fitness journey is not about you, saints. It's not about food or exercise or recipes or push-ups. It's about glorifying God by caring for the home of the Holy Spirit, admitting your inability, and acknowledging the immeasurable riches of His grace and celebrating His mercy by revering His masterpiece. Never forget that.

Earlier we looked at George Muller's undaunted commitment to prayer, relying solely on God to bless his ministry to orphans while remaining debt-free. His higher purpose, though, was to reveal God's presence and goodness to other believers. He observed a weakness in faith in the Church, not unlike today, and desperately wanted to model unrestricted reliance upon the Lord.

"Blessed to be a blessing," is a familiar expression. Though commonly interpreted in financial terms, let's look at George Muller's faith model. He never asked for money and never went into debt because he was intent upon giving God *all* the glory. He knew he couldn't accomplish what he did without divine grace. As my heart slowly softens, absolutely exclusively by His grace, He will be glorified. When people begin to ask how you achieved such dramatic physical improvement, won't it be gratifying to tell them it was all by God's goodness and mercy?

There are rare stories about someone down in the dregs, addicted to alcohol, drugs, an illegal and perverse business, who was immediately and fully transformed after committing his life to Jesus. Most Christians don't have that speedy, life-altering conversion. But remember, we *are* called to be set apart, *distinct* from the world. Sanctification is a slow, arduous, roller-coaster journey.

A personal floating device (PFD), more commonly known as a life jacket, keeps non-swimmers afloat. Following are two spiritual pfd's for your regular reference. Convert into confessions.

[11]*To this end we always pray for you, that our God may make you worthy of his calling and may fulfill every resolve for good and every work of faith by his power,* [12]*so that the name of our Lord Jesus may be glorified in you, and you in him, according to the grace of our God and the Lord Jesus Christ* (2 Thessalonians 1:11-12).

[20]*Now to him who is able to do far more abundantly than all that we ask or think, according to the power at work within us,* [21]*to him be glory in the church and in Christ Jesus throughout all generations, forever and ever. Amen* (Ephesians 3:20-21).

With Thanksgiving

Oh give thanks to the LORD, for he is good, for his steadfast love endures forever! (Psalm 107:1)

Much has been made of the power of gratitude. It elevates your spirit and lowers your blood pressure. It lifts your thoughts and attitudes. Gratitude softens your heart.

We all can be cross. From unexpected expenses to annoying humans, every day throws us bad mood barbs. But gratitude is a barb buster. It shatters the venomous arrows that can instantly turn me and you into the Wicked Witch. Instead, sweet Glinda stands strong. (Are you lost? Brush up on your Fairy Tales.

https://www.youtube.com/watch?v=TP_wx0qrKu0)

Jesus' mother, Mary, personifies gratefulness. She was privileged to be chosen to birth the promised Messiah. Yet when the angel appeared to convey the news, it wasn't tantamount to Publishers Clearing House on the front porch filming the thrilling moment. A young virgin girl suspiciously showing up pregnant created complications, especially with her fiancé, Joseph. "Honestly, Joe . . ." But did she fret or complain? Hardly. Read her prayer in Luke 1, then consider all God has done for you. Even if your current circumstances are confusing, pause and pray Luke 1:46-49 for yourself.

Are you grateful to be on this new health journey? For the bounty of God-grown foods that are abundantly available to you? That you have a miraculous body that serves you well, even if you haven't always returned the favor? Take a moment and give God thanks.

_____

_____

_____

Eyes on the Prize

forgetting what lies behind and straining forward to what lies ahead, I press on toward the goal for the prize of the upward call of God in Christ Jesus (Philippians 3:13-14).

Embrace grace. Whether your personal aspiration is to improve your fitness, banish your anger, or simply be a better image-bearer, sanctification unfolds solely by His grace. Eating and drinking and doing all that you do for the glory of God is a tough challenge. You must abide in the Vine. When you trip and fall, He will gently pick you up and whisper, "Don't worry. You will learn from this. Your eyes strayed from Me." He helps you up and brushes you off. "Let's try this again. Let me hold your hand. I will strengthen you. I will help you. I will uphold you with my righteous right hand."

Thoughts?

_____

_____

_____

_____

_____

_____

Kept

As I slowly opened my heart to God helping me to better surrender, I came upon the word kept.

kept – tend, care for, provide for, support, sustain, protect, guard, defend, safeguard, nurture

Every word grabbed me. Like Christmas time with a bounty of gifts beneath the tree, it was all I ever yearned for. Protection. Support. Care.

I plunged into the Word for references to "kept."

Now may the God of peace Himself sanctify you completely, and may your whole spirit and soul and body be kept *blameless at the coming of our Lord Jesus Christ. He who calls you is faithful. He will surely do it* (1 Thessalonians 5:23-24).

Sit with those last two statements for a moment. *He who calls you is faithful. He will surely do it.* He will keep you. Write it on your heart.

When Jesus prayed in John 17, He asked His Father to *keep them in Your name* (John 17:11). Keep means to tend or care for; to cause to continue without change; to restrain or prevent; (vt) to remain unchanged. So, Jesus was petitioning God to continually hold us tightly in His name.

Kept was my new favorite word.

One of my cherished family treasures is a book entitled *Kept for the Master's Use*, by Frances Ridley Havergal, copyright 1895. She prays, " . . . by His grace, may we enter upon a new era of experience, our lives kept for Him more fully than ever before, because we trust Him more simply and unreservedly to keep them."

I was all in for entering into a new era of experience of being provided for, supported, safeguarded, and nurtured.

But Miss Frances threw me a curve.

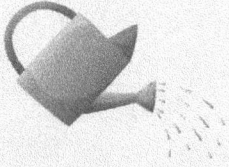

Judi's Journal 7/29/15

Kept for the Master's Use, Frances Ridley Havergal

✓ Kept for His sake
✓ Kept for His use
✓ Kept to be His witness
✓ Kept for His joy
✓ Kept to do His will and His work in His own way
✓ Kept, maybe to suffer, for His sake
✓ Kept that He may do just what seemeth Him good with me
✓ Kept, so no other Lord shall have dominion over me

And when we waver from His purpose for keeping us, she asks:

"Day after day passes on, and year after year, and what shall your harvest be? What is your present return? Are you getting any real and lasting satisfaction out of it all?"

Lord, I confess that when you first gave me Ms. Havergal's words, I leapt for joy and shouted, "Yes! I want to be kept!" I want to be protected, provided for, safe, comfortable. All along ignoring the last four words, "for the Master's use."

You don't keep me for my comfort – my recognition – my financial security. You keep me – heal me – protect me – love me – THAT I MIGHT GO DO THE SAME.

Seems being kept by Jesus isn't all about me. Havergal suggests I am kept for His sake, His use, His witness. Kept for His glory. Kept to be a keeper. Blessed to be a blessing (Proverbs 11:25-26).

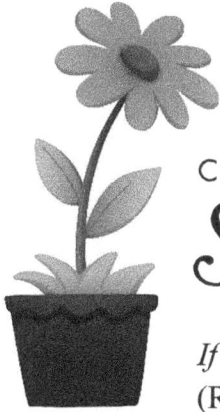

CHAPTER 11
Share The Good News

If we hope for what we do not yet have, we wait for it patiently
(Romans 8:25).

Hope upholds. God's Word has opened your eyes to His grace. His power is perfected in your weakness. You can have absolute faith that surrendering to the Spirit transforms you from the inside out (Romans 7-8). He who is doing a good work in you will continue to perfect it until the day of Christ (Philippians 1:6). You have cast the burden of unhealthy temptations on Him (1 Peter 5:7). He has given your heart new desires (Psalm 37:4). You are no longer a slave to former desires of the flesh (Romans 6:6). You are free indeed (John 8:36). Don't you want to shout this great news from the housetops?

One of our many callings in Christ is building one another up. For our Church family members who feel physically defeated by excess weight, depleted energy, and/or debilitating disease, shall we not also uplift them physically? Support someone today by suggesting a walk together, share a simple, healthy recipe, or by giving them a fitness ball vs. a birthday cake.

Nobody understands the benefits of the Buddy System better than Christians. *For where two or three are gathered in my name, there shall I be in their midst* (Matthew 18:20). Our commitment to doing life together strengthens our faith, growth, and service. *Though one may be overpowered, two can defend themselves. A cord of three strands is not quickly broken* (Ecclesiastes 4:12).

And so it is with our physical fitness. We are much more likely to stand up and stretch, avoid that unhelpful treat, or go to that Zumba class if we're accountable to a friend. The good news is the call to physical stewardship can easily be incorporated into our routines. Walk with your buddies instead of meeting for coffee. (And pie?) When your small group gathers, ask all to share their successes and prayer requests in their food and exercise intentions. Serve wholesome snacks. Commit to encouraging and spurring one another in caring for the most magnificent of physical gifts, our bodies. For as the Church inspires each other, we can be the light on the hill for others.

Who do you know who would feel loved and supported if you invited them for a weekly walk, committed to an exercise class with them, or taught them easy, healthy cooking tips? Support someone else and fuel your own success. Experience the magic of inner transformation by uplifting another.

Beloved, let us love one another, for love is from God, and whoever loves has been born of God and knows God (1 John 4:7).

And that is the purpose of HolyHealthClub.com. It's a place for Christians to stir one another up to eat real food and take long walks, based on the truth of the Word. Come join us, and be sure to bring your friends with you.

Then stand up and sing with alacrity the stirring song from Godspell:

https://www.youtube.com/watch?v=zg4GOgZ-L1I

A Challenge to the Church

Should we be concerned by the poor physical condition of so many believers? Will we continue to close our eyes to obesity and infirmity in the Body of Christ? According to Dr. Golubic of the Cleveland Clinic, "About 80% of chronic diseases are driven by lifestyle factors such as diet and exercise." [https://health.clevelandclinic.org/5-healthy-habits-that-prevent-chronic-disease/] It's time to take seriously this startling statistic and begin encouraging one another in our physical self-care, including rethinking the foods we serve at our godly gatherings. So I challenge the Church: Take 10 minutes at every small group meeting to invite members to share their physical concerns, aspirations, intentions and progress. Commit to exhort one another physically as well as spiritually. In addition, begin a conversation at your church about after-service snacks, rethinking how you can better love the Body.

Then consider the terrific opportunity for ministry. A huge percentage of Americans struggle with their food, weight, and well-being. They may think it's about spinach and strength training, but what you now know is it's all about the redeeming grace of Jesus the Christ. What if you invited non-Christians into your conversation? It could lead them to abundant life, today and forever.

We are not our own, Church. We have been bought with a price. Let's glorify God in our body and in our spirit, which are God's.

Now to Him who is able to keep you from stumbling and to present you blameless before the presence of His glory with great joy, to the only God, our Savior, through Jesus Christ our Lord, be glory, majesty, dominion, and authority, before all time and now and forever. Amen. (Jude 24-25)

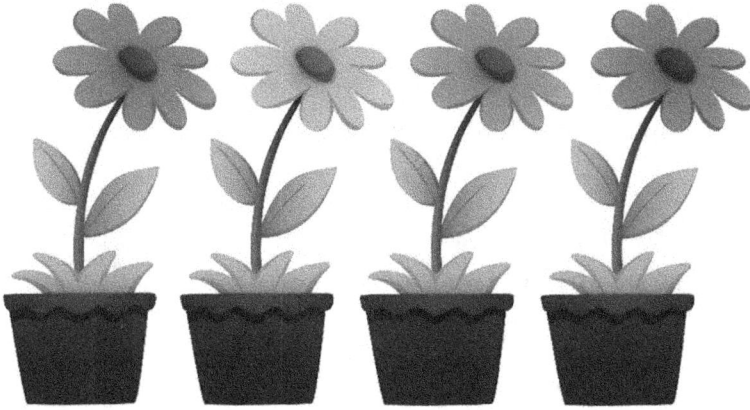

Welcome to the Lab

Do you remember eighth grade science class, when the lectures were complemented by a weekly, hands-on lab? From dissecting frogs to viewing worlds unknown in petri dishes and turning test tubes into mini-volcanos, the purpose was to transform head knowledge into memorable experiences. That's the intent of this section; it's your lab work. You will use the spiritual principles in Part 1 to make physical practices a reality.

So, whether you eat or drink, or whatever you do, do all to the glory of God (1 Corinthians 10:31).

May this be your mantra. Note, it's preceded by 1 Corinthians 6:12 and 10:23 that we considered when determining your deep-down WHY. *All things are lawful for me, but not all things are helpful. All things are lawful for me, but I will not be dominated by anything. All things are lawful, but not all things are helpful. All things are lawful, but not all things build up.* Was Paul running out of things to say, or was he purposely emphasizing his point? I'm guessing the latter, which means we should take note.

Is this the first time you've started a fitness program by asking yourself whether your food, beverages, and body movement glorifies God? Making conscientious choices vs. merely succumbing to a dominating internal desire? This perspective sets the table differently, doesn't it?

In my thirty-plus years of health promotion, only once did I do personal training. As I sat in the office of the Human Resources Director of a large real estate development company, trying to convince him of the benefits of an employee wellness program, he said, "I'm the one who needs a wellness program." Spontaneously I replied, "Let me train you." That was the beginning of many months of hard work, great fun, and much progress for Mr. D who remains a good friend.

Are you ready for me to be your personal trainer? I warn you, I'm tough. You'd best be prepared to sacrifice and sweat. But as Mr. D would attest, in addition to being difficult and sometimes frustrating, it will also be rewarding and fun.

At the risk of offending anyone, it seems analogous to our call to follow Christ. *Truly, truly, I say to you, unless a grain of wheat falls into the earth and dies, it remains alone; but if it dies, it bears much fruit* (John 12:24). "Truly, truly" means pay attention, this is important. Has the church been willing to die to self, both spiritually *and* physically? The statistics in the introduction offer insight.

Now's your chance! It's time for you to get into the game, putting God's promises into practice. But here's the catch: You shouldn't go it alone. As stated early in the book, just like our call to engage with the Church community, the journey of self-care is best trod hand-in-hand. All the 10:31 Habits (1 Corinthians 10:31) presented below are to be done with a friend. Or . . . what a great opportunity to spend time with someone who doesn't know our Lord.

An Honest Assessment

Before you suit up, let's pinpoint your starting place. You can't map your course unless you know where you are, right? So, pull out your pen and muse a moment on what prompted you to dive into this ever-niggling issue. Be specific. The more clearly you assess and address your weaknesses the more productive your time investment will be. How would you like your life to look different 3, 6, 12 months from now?

Your Faith:

Do you take time daily to be in the Word and listen for the Lord's voice?

_____

Do you seek scriptures to address your concerns? Do you regularly recite and memorize them?

_____

_____

Would you describe your prayer habits as earnest or fervent? *The fervent prayers of a righteous man accomplish much* (James 5:16).

_____

Are you actively engaged in open, honest, vulnerable and accountable Christian relationships?

_____

Your Food:

Are most of your foods given or grown by God (i.e. unprocessed, not boxed)?
Watch this video: https://vimeo.com/127372876

Do you start most days with a nutritious breakfast?

_____

What's hiding in your healthy snack stash at work?

_____

Three hours before bedtime, do you STOP eating?

_____

How many fruits or veggies do you consume most days? Five or more?

_____

Your Fitness:

Are you active at least 30 minutes most days? How often do you huff and puff vs. lollygag?

_____

Watch this video, then note what thoughts emerge: https://vimeo.com/105381209

_____

_____

If you are a daily desk-sitter, do you stand up and move a few minutes every hour?

_____

What's your strength training regimen?

_____

Do you schedule times of quiet relaxation every day? If not, why not?

_____

Is God speaking to you about your fitness? What is He saying? How do you want to respond?

_____

Your Figures:

How many times a week do you weigh yourself? Do your moods move in sync with the scale?

_____

Have you ever had your body fat tested? Do you know what that is?

_____

How do you assess whether your heart is getting stronger?

_____

If your goal is to gain muscle, how will you gauge?

_____

When was the last time you had a blood test?

_____

Most people rely solely on scale weight to rate improvement, but we'll be offering other alternatives for celebrating success.

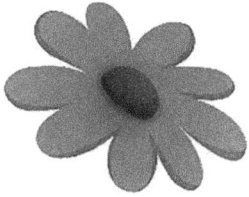

LAB 1

Focus On Fitness

I remember decades ago the wellness world began to soften the call to fitness. They quit using the word exercise because it sounded too harsh, and instead encouraged "moving." Well guess what gang, anything worthwhile requires discipline and resolve, and you betcha, sometimes it's hard. The idea that everyone in the race gets a trophy regardless of their performance is a destructive and demeaning fallacy. We're going to focus on fitness.

As we consider the importance of a variety of statistics, let's start with a quote by a Cleveland Clinic physician, Dr. Stanley Hazen: "Cardiovascular disease is the leading cause of death in the United States, killing over 1 million Americans each year." https://my.clevelandclinic.org/departments/heart/patient-education/webchats/prevention/20030_cardiovascular-disease-risk-factors-primary-and-secondary-prevention

Though we look forward to eternity with our Lord Jesus, you're probably not quite ready to enter the pearly gates. A few risk factors for heart disease are beyond our control – age (older), gender (men higher risk), family history, postmenopausal women, and non-whites. There are a number of *controllable* risk factors, though, that are rampant within the church community.

- Hypertension (high blood pressure)
- High HDL and low LDL/VLDL cholesterol levels
- High C-reactive protein
- Uncontrolled diabetes
- Obesity (BMI above 25)
- Stress, anger, and/or depression
- Physical inactivity
- Poor diet
- Alcohol abuse
- Smoking

How many do you have? You *don't* want a perfect score on this one. _____

Most of these are straightforward, so we won't discuss, but a few words on a handful.

147

Blood Pressure

They call it the silent killer. The widow maker. Hypertension is a *big* deal, folks, and many people have it and don't even know it, because they're generally asymptomatic. But elevated blood pressure raises your risk of suffering a heart attack or stroke.

As you likely know, blood pressure includes two numbers. The first, or systolic, is the pressure in your arteries when your heart is beating. It increases with stress, activity, and age. The second number, or diastolic, is the arterial pressure between heart beats. It is measured in mm/Hg, referring to the height to which the pressure in the blood vessels push a column of mercury. (You remember Hg as mercury from chemistry class, right?) Though many focus primarily on the diastolic, people over the age of 65 are especially susceptible to elevated systolic pressure (over 130), which should be watched and addressed with your doctor.

The statistics below reveal the progression of hypertension according to the Mayo Clinic:

Systolic *OR* Diastolic

Elevated blood pressure 120-129 mm Hg < 80 mm Hg
Stage 1 hypertension 130-139 mm Hg 80 to 89 mm Hg
Stage 2 hypertension 140 mm Hg or higher 90 mm Hg or higher.

Again, let's look at controllable* risk factors:

- excess dietary salt (i.e. processed and restaurant foods)
- insufficient potassium
- inactivity
- chronic stress
- smoking
- excess alcohol

Do you know your blood pressure? It's a need-to-know, so go find a machine at your local pharmacy. And won't it be fun to watch it drop as you increase your activity?

Cholesterol

H is for happy; remember that when you're looking at your cholesterol results. HDL, or high-density lipoproteins, are the "good" guys, because they reduce risk of heart

---

* You can lower your blood pressure by changing your habits.

disease. LDL (low-density lipoproteins) and VLDL (very low-density) are the "bad boys," primarily because they contribute to plaque buildup in your arteries, increasing your risk of a heart attack. Like the Lone Ranger, your HDL cholesterol rounds up the bad guys, and even recycles, transporting the unwanted waste to the liver to be reprocessed. HDL also scrubs the mess made by LDL inside your blood vessels, further reducing your risk of heart attack or stroke. Ideally, HDL should be at least one third of your total, indicated by your risk ratio, which is total cholesterol divided by HDL. The higher your HDL, the lower your risk ratio, which is better. Check out these examples:

Total HDL Risk Ratio

200 25 8
200 50 4
200 100 2

In 10:31 Habit #6 you'll be listing the pros and cons of exercise. Be sure to add this to the plus side.

Additionally, and/or alternatively, you may want to consider checking your C-reactive protein (CRP) which indicates inflammation in the arteries. CRP is one of the proteins produced by the liver to heal the LDL cholesterol's damage to arterial walls.

Body Fat Percentage

I'm betting you know your weight, but do you know your body fat percentage? Do you know what that is and why it's important?

Your total weight is irrelevant because it has two contributors. Lean weight, from your bones, muscles, organs, and body fluids, should be about 75% of a woman's total weight, and 85% for men. Experts calculate it backwards, focusing on percentage of fat to total weight. So, backing out of the previous recommendations, women should carry no more than 25% fat, and men 15%. American's aren't big on following the rules, and this advice is no exception. According to the U.S. Centers for Disease Control and Prevention's National Center for Health Statistics, American women hover around 40% and men are bulging at 28%. (https://www.livestrong.com/article/380221-national-body-fat-percentage-average/) As a population, we're over fat. But the scale doesn't differentiate! Go on a crazy starvation diet, surviving on carrots and celery (and an occasional binge . . .), and you likely will lose muscle, not fat.

Parents be aware: Kids are getting fatter. The statistics are staggering. What was once referred to as "adult onset diabetes" is now being diagnosed in children. Overweight kids are far more likely to become obese adults. It is imperative parents understand this important fact: obesity is determined by a person's total number of fat cells, and their size. Cell size varies throughout life, but *the number of fat cells is determined in childhood, and remains unchanged after adolescence.* Children who eat poorly and exercise rarely will develop an unnecessary number of fat cells, making it very difficult to manage their weight the rest of their lives.

So how do I measure my body fat?

Hydrostatic, or under water weighing, is considered by many the most accurate means of measuring body fat. Because fat is less dense than water, it floats; lean is heavier, so it sinks. Based on the Archimedes theory of displacement, only lean weight displaces water when you submerge. In a hydrostatic weighing tank, after expelling as much air from your lungs as possible and "dunking", the weight is entered into a complicated computation and voila, you know your body fat. A local community college or university may be your best bet for finding a tank, though in some regions you may find a mobile testing unit, like Fitness Wave. (www.getdunked.com) Don't forget to bring your bathing suit!

Skinfold calipers are also popular, and much more readily accessible and affordable. A consultant will "pinch an inch" of fat at 3-7 different body locations measuring the thickness of the fat underneath skin (subcutaneous). From there they use a fancy formula to calculate body fat percentage. Many health clubs offer skin caliper testing.

Technically known as Air Displacement Plethysmography, the Bod Pod uses the same principals of displacement as hydrostatic weighing, but it's moving air rather than water. It's also easier than getting dunked in a tank because you sit in an egg-shaped chamber and simply wait for the air to be displaced and the verdict to pop out. Though the results are quite accurate, unfortunately, if you can find a Bod Pod it will likely be pricey.

If you want to dish out some dough, look into a Dual-Energy X-ray Absorptiometry (DXA) scan. As the name suggests, it's an x-ray technology that not only differentiates between lean and fat weight, it can calculate by body regions. So, if you're a cyclist and want to track how beefy your leg muscles are getting, a DXA will tell you. Another advantage is it determines bone density, an important statistic to track, especially for women. The big hurdle to DXA is accessibility and expense, as it's normally only available in medical facilities.

Some gyms still offer bio-electrical impedance. I wouldn't waste my money.

The message is punt your scale. Begin concentrating on your lean/fat weight ratio.

Watch this video about body fat testing: https://vimeo.com/45798798

My friend Kim Taylor refers to hyper-focus on scale weight as "scale worship." A bit harsh, but I have known many people who base their feelings and faith on the morning number coming from the box on the bathroom floor. Have you been lured into that trap? Is there an inverse correlation between your weight and your mood? Remember, the scale provides incomplete information. Listen to this session on Stirring Words: https://www.holyhealthclub.com/new-blog/2020/9/30/get-off-the-scale

Other important figures

Since we focused so intensely on issues of the spiritual heart in Part 1, let's now focus on our physical heart. Is strengthening your cardiovascular system one of your goals? How will you quantify improvements? Actually, it's a fingertip away. The stronger your heart is, the more blood it drives through your system with every beat, so your heart rate is lower. Unlike our philosophy of life, slower is better. Resting heart rate is the number of times your heart beats per minute when you're resting. Not when you're stressed. Not when you've just dodged a traffic accident. When life is calm. So, the best time to check is when you first wake up in the morning. Let's check it now, the old -fashioned way:

Touch both your index and middle fingers either on your wrist, along your thumb line, or on one of your two carotid arteries in your neck. Be careful, it's the blood's pipeline to your brain; you could pass out if you press too hard.

Feel it? Now count for 15 seconds, then multiply that number by 4. That's your resting heart rate.

Here's a demo. https://www.youtube.com/watch?v=bB7j0lvso7Q

You may choose to use an activity tracker, smartwatch, your phone, or other heart rate monitor to track your ticker. It's all good. The point is, check it. Get into the habit of logging it every morning. The more consistent your exercise, the lower your pulse. Celebrate progress.

Note: What does it mean if your morning heart rate normally averages around 60 bpm (beats per minute), and one day you awaken to a rat-a-tat 80? Your body is stressed from over-training, illness, or a troubled spirit. It's requesting rest. Please listen.

Watching your recovery rate is another important cardiovascular fitness test, but *only do this if you have been exercising awhile and do not have a heart condition.* The stronger your heart is, the more quickly it will recover being elevated. Get out and do your normal aerobic exercise. Walk. Run. Ride a stationary bike. Get your pumper revved a bit, and note the number, ideally using a heart rate monitor. (There are exceptions, but for safety's sake, don't go above 150 bpm.) Then slow 'er down. *Do not stop*, but walk or ride more slowly. After three minutes, take your heart rate again. Have you recovered to 120 bpm? 90? You're back down to 60 bpm? As you track from week to week, watch your recovery rate improve. Go get 'em!

VO2

VO2 is the volume of oxygen your heart can distribute through your system during exercise. The stronger it is, the more air is delivered. Typically, VO2 is determined by a graded exercise test on a calibrated treadmill or bicycle. The clinician notes the participant's heart rate at gradually increasing workloads. If a light load drastically elevates the person's heartrate, his cardiovascular condition is poor. Conversely, if it takes a tough exertion to nudge his pulse into the targeted exercise zone, his heart efficiently, effectively, and powerfully moves oxygen to the muscles in need.

What if, instead of focusing solely on weight loss, you set specific cardiovascular goals? Wouldn't your friends be surprised (and encouraged), when you told them your secret to success was heart strength! There's an analogy hiding in there, don't you think? When your heart is transformed from stone to flesh, so you are surrendered to God's will and His Word, you will enthusiastically tend to your temple, and your heart becomes hardy. A new heart begets a new heart.

Watch this video on measuring cardiovascular fitness: https://vimeo.com/45672926

Strength and Flexibility

Though strength and flexibility testing are a bit primitive, monitoring is better than not monitoring.

If you currently never stretch, can't touch your toes, you start stretching and within eight weeks can extend two inches beyond your toes, isn't that significant? But you would never know you progressed unless you kept track.

Sometimes consultants use a sit-and-reach box to measure flexibility. It is literally a yardstick-on-a-box. You can make your ow by . . . gluing a yardstick on a box. Place your feet on the side of the box and with one hand atop the other, fingers aligned, slowly bend forward moving your hands along the yardstick. How many inches can you reach? Watch your progress, but remember, don't push!

The same goes for strength testing. If today you can barely do one full push up, but over a period of time you improve to ten, you're building your buff, right? And if you can only "stomach" ten crunches* when you start your program, and slowly advance to a hundred every day, your abs are abs-solutely getting stronger.

Keep tabs. It is motivational and inspirational. And more reasons to celebrate.

Fitness Record

Appendix 4 offers a Fitness Record on which you can make entries of blood pressure, resting heart rate, recovery rate, push-ups, sit-ups and sit-and-reach. (The weight entry is optional.)

Keeping this log current will give you a format for regularly monitoring your physical progress in all the key areas. Keeping track keeps you on track!

P.A.S.S.

Remember the KISS principle: Keep it simple, silly. (Kindness honored here.) Alongside the spirit-stirring conversation in Part 1 about God's sovereignty & grace, counterfeit gods, surrender, and sanctification, we're going to introduce specific action steps. As you begin to embrace the guidelines and habits provided, focus on the PASS process:

Pray – Don't even think about beginning before you commit your way to the Lord.

Admit – Confess you can't on your own accord, and admit when you falter.

Surrender – Let God lead. Ask Him to sprinkle you with clean water. Trust His power to perfect your weakness.

---

* Never do the old-fashioned full sit-up. Instead, with your hands supporting your head, look up to the ceiling and *using your abdominal muscles*, raise your shoulders 4-6 inches off the ground.

Share – Support someone else. Encourage others to move often and fuel well. Uplift a sister with scripture. The more you give away the redeeming power of the Word, the deeper your sanctification.

Here we go!

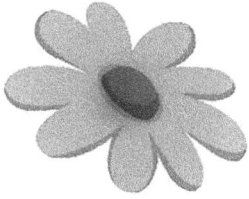

LAB 2
Eat Real Food

Food controversy abounds. There are those who think carbs are the tool of the devil, and others say meat is the monster. And of course, both claim to be "evidenced-based," evaluated by doctors. Who do you believe?

We're going to consider several specific eating guidelines in our 10:31 Habits, but the overriding principal is **Eat Real Food**. Consider the difference between fresh fruit and Froot Loops. Corn and corn chips, especially flavored. A bowl of oatmeal and an oatmeal cookie. How would you differentiate the formers from the latters? Fruit, corn, and oatmeal are God-made, real food; the others fabricated. Given our discussion in Part 1 of counterfeit comforts, it seems logical to ponder fake foods. What do you consider "food"? Does it include anything and everything available? Are there guiding principles by which you choose? Like our misguided images of the Almighty, it's easy to accept imposter sustenance; temptations that don't satisfy. Take for example, those items whose ingredients list consume a ton of real estate on the package. Have you ever taken the time (and it will take a minute) to read the ingredients list for Cheese Whiz? Question: If there are words you can't pronounce, is it still food? Many seem befuddled about how to improve their diet. There's some consensus that colas are "bad" and carrots are "good," but are you really limited to tofu and greens?

Emphatically "No!"

One of the easiest ways to assess an option is by asking, "Is this unprocessed, God-grown or given?"

Watch this video: https://vimeo.com/75725516

I promise, banning fake foods won't leave your tumbly grumbling. Consider the plethora of options offering appetizing nourishment:

Fruits & veggies – Have you considered lately the wealth of choices God has given in the produce department? Take a peek at Appendix 1. What percentage of the list do you regularly consume? Savored a kiwi lately?

Lean proteins – People put a premium on protein, and mostly think of meats, but you have a handful of luscious sources:

- Meats – Balance your burgers with a bird and a fish.
- Beans – According to the Center for Disease Control, there are "hundreds of varieties of beans" so boredom should never be a problem. Start the Bean-a-Week Club with your friends! (Don't go there; fart prattle is impolite.)
- Nuts and seeds – Explore beyond dry roasted peanuts. Walnuts, pecans, and hazelnuts are great sources for anti-inflammatory Omega 3 fatty acids which reduce risk of heart disease and stroke, joint pain and depression. Chia and flaxseeds are O-3 loaded too, so be sure to grind and sprinkle on anything and everything. "Could you pass the salt, pepper, and chia, please?"
- Dairy – Though naturally high in calcium, some discourage dairy consumption. If you do indulge, go with reduced-fat renditions, though watch for added sugar. And remember, cottage cheese is more prudent than Rocky Road.

Whole grains – As mentioned above, carbs are controversial. Many avoid them like exercise. But not all carbohydrates are created equal, and not all peeps have the same internal reaction to them.

Watch this video: https://vimeo.com/125092492

As we focus on eating real food, your best complex carbohydrate bites are whole grains. A grain of wheat, like what Jesus got in trouble for picking, is composed of three parts. Like an egg, the bran is the outer shell that protects the inner seed. Though it's full of helpful insoluble fiber, it's all too often discarded. The largest part of the inner seed is the endosperm which is the primary ingredient from which white flour is made. But the germ, or the sprouting section, is the smaller portion that contains the most nutrients, including antioxidants, vitamins E and B, protein, minerals, and oils. Now you under-stand why eating highly processed breads and crackers cheat you out of valuable nourishment. Instead, cook some quinoa.

Note that complex carbohydrates are converted to glucose which your body uses for fuel. You need go juice to keep you moving during your days; not so much before bedtime. So, though they are an important part of a healthy food plan, it's smart to cut back after lunch. Create colorful protein and veggie combos for supper.

We get stuck in the white rice rut, thinking brown takes too long to cook. Did you know quinoa and millet are ready in just 10-15 minutes?

How would you rate your grain repertoire?

_____

Salsas, Sauces, Spices & Dressings – This is the category that tantalizes your taste buds. What's your pleasure? Hot & spicy? Sweet, yet sassy? Mexican? Thai? Teriyaki? Spices and salsas bring your bowl to life.

Maybe your cooking confusion is creating tasty combos. Clearly naked quinoa is less than alluring. Simply choose one or more ingredients from each category above according to your mood. Add a little of this and a bit of that and presto-chango, dinner is served.

Watch this video: https://vimeo.com/77003191

Tips:

1. Always have a tub o' grains already cooked so you're ready to throw in your bowl and go.
2. Try cooking your morning grain in ¼ C OJ and ¾ C. water. Gives it a sweet citrus flavor.
3. Chopping veggies in advance saves some time, but will expedite spoilage. Prep ahead only a few days.
4. Teach your children well. This is a great opportunity to involve your kids in your meals. Ask them to choose something from each category, allowing them to be creative in their mix & match.

Remember to over-prep for dinner so you have leftovers for tomorrow's lunchboxes.

Here are more ideas to prime your culinary pump:

- Diced and sautéed onion, peppers, sweet potato, and black beans, topped with avocado and your favorite salsa
- Stir-fry a medley of veggies, add diced chicken, brown and wild rice (from your tub of ready-made in the fridge), and Teriyaki sauce (low sodium please).
- Quinoa, garbanzo beans (chickpeas), sunflower seeds, chopped spinach and arugula, diced red peppers, halved cherry tomatoes topped with vinaigrette dressing. This is a GREAT lunchbox item.
- Breakfast – Whatever's in your tub o' grains, chopped walnuts, berries and a bit o' organic sugar in that dollop of plain Greek yogurt.

Though it may feel a little daunting, it's actually pretty easy to whip up your own salad dressing. Your basic ingredient is usually extra virgin olive oil, oftentimes balsamic vinegar, sometimes OJ and orange zest, and maybe lime, ground mustard, and many times, garlic. Google it, girl!

But what if you have a hankering for a packaged snack? It's game time and only chips and salsa will do. Read before you feed. Be leery of lengthy labels. Compare the ingredients of two brands of corn chips:

> Option #1: Stone ground white corn, sunflower oil or corn oil (Do they decide by what's on sale?), sea salt, water, trace of Lime.

> Option #2: Whole corn, vegetable oil (sunflower, canola, corn, and/or soybean oil), maltodextrin (made from corn), and less than 2% of the following: wheat flour, salt, cheddar cheese (milk, cheese cultures, salt, enzymes), whey, monosodium glutamate, buttermilk, Romano cheese (part-skim cow's milk, cheese cultures, salt, enzymes), whey protein concentrate, onion powder, partially hydrogenated soybean and cottonseed oil, corn flour, natural and artificial flavor, dextrose, tomato powder, lactose, spices, artificial color (including yellow 6, yellow 5, red 40), lactic acid, citric acid, sugar, garlic powder, skim milk, whey protein isolate, corn syrup solids, red and green bell pepper powder, sodium caseinate, disodium inosinate, and disodium guanylate. Whew! These names even confused spell-check!

Which seems the most sensible?

As you ponder your platter, choose real foods.

Get Out of the Box

In the 1950's, many began planning meals out of convenience vs. nutritional value. We slowly slipped from boiling macaroni noodles, adding milk and cheese, to grabbing the Kraft box, complete with bright orange powder. Rather than mixing flour, milk, eggs, etc. for the morning pancake feed we let Aunt Jemima do most of the work. Not only is the experience diluted, so are the nutrients.

Watch this video: https://vimeo.com/38933311

The Pantry Purge

The words of a dog trainer I hired for an unruly hound have stuck with me for years: "Your job is to keep Jackson out of trouble." What he was suggesting was, Jackson can't eat the plumber if he's in down dog. Similarly, you can't eat the ice cream if it isn't in your freezer. (I wonder how many gallons of Breyers* are sold across America after 9 p.m.?) Following simple, supportive systems make life a lot easier. It stops the internal debate. It brings clarity. It can even become a game with your kids.

Start with controlling your environment. Purging, then preparing your pantry are the best first steps to bolster your self-control. Let's start with the hardest: purging. If Oprah Winfrey and her camera crew were to show up at your front door to video your fridge and pantry for a future show, how would you feel? (Never mind the mess in the living room . . .)

You're in this to win this, right? You're ready to kick some unhealthy habits to the curb, correct? OK, take a deep breath, hug your kitty if necessary, go grab a big, black garbage bag, and throw out any of these that are in your house or office: chips, boxed anything, cookies/candy/cakes, scary colored snacks (orange, puffy worm-like things). *Don't even think* about whispering "I won't buy any more after these are gone." Go on. You have some purging to do.

Next, stock what you want to eat. You can't snack on veggies and hummus while you're prepping supper if you got no hummus. Given our food formula of heavy veggie + lean protein + whole grains = happy body, what's conspicuously missing in your fridge and pantry?

See Appendix 3 for a shopping list. Note: This isn't exhaustive or necessarily a perfect fit for everyone. It's simply meant to get your real food juices flowing.

P.A.S.S.

Pray to be enlightened on what would be considered Real Food.

Admit to your Father your fondness for destructive foods.

Surrender your nagging desires for immediate gratification, asking for divine strength.

Share and discuss the idea of eating "real food" with someone near, or far.

---

* Did you know Breyers has been around since 1866? Americans love ice cream!

Fitness Focus:

1. What fabricated foods are your favorite? What alternatives can you consider?

   _____

   _____

2. What boxed products reside in your pantry? What's your next right step of improvement?

   _____

   _____

3. What scripture will you claim this week when you start to crave potato chips?

   _____

4. How would you like your friend/small group to support you?

   _____

The Big 10
(A fond phrase for an Indiana Hoosier)

Just as there are specific spiritual disciplines that enhance your relationship with God, there are also physical disciplines that sustain health. There are definitely discrepancies, discussions and dissent in the food arena, but on several healthy habits everyone agrees. Since your personal library is packed with diet and exercise books and DVDs (reveals how long you've had them . . .), you can undoubtedly list them yourself. With the help of hints, can you name the universal recommendations?

1. Two guidelines in this one.

   1) Eating from a salad plate prompts you to _____ .

   2) A 1950's divided dinner plate erroneously guides you to _____ .

Here's some help:

   https://vimeo.com/77517222

2. _____ is your most important meal.

3. They're quite colorful and we're called to eat 9-a-day.

   _____

4. It has a variety of names, colas are full of it, and it is an enticement regularly offered after church.

   _____

5. It's that time of day you want to eat most and need to least. It's a temptation often associated with late night TV.

   _____

6. Folks do it differently – walking, cycling, hiking, playing pickleball – and the recommendation is 30 minutes a day.

   _____

7. Arnold Schwarzenegger is known for his. Use 'em or lose 'em.

   _____

8. Dogs do it during their lazy days, but we only think about it before exercise. It's football players' pre-game ritual.

   _____

9. The earth is mostly covered with it, and you can lead a horse to it.

   _____

10. A lost art in today's frenetic society. Could include a comfy comforter and a good book, an afternoon siesta, or a walk in the woods.

   _____

How did you do? Below is our 10:31 Healthy Habits* checklist:

1. Size up your plate (portion size & plate proportions)
2. Fuel Early (Eat Breakfast)
3. Think Color
4. Shun Sugar
5. STOP! Eating
6. *MOVE!* Often
7. Strength Training
8. S-T-R-E-T-C-H
9. Drink Up
10. Rest Regularly

---

* If you have attempted though fizzled in sticking to these habits before, the game-changer this time will be considering each in the context of 1 Corinthians 10:31: *So, whether you eat or drink, or whatever you do, do all to the glory of God.* Living for His glory supplies inviolable inspiration!

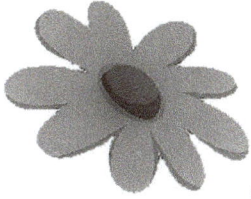

LAB 3
10:31 HABIT #1:

Size Up Your Servings

The fruit of the Spirit is love, joy, peace, patience . . . and self-control (Galatians 5:22-23).

"Let's say grace." Why is a short prayer of gratitude uplifted before meals called grace? How many bow before eating these days? Sadly, many families no longer gather for supper. Assuming you say grace, what do you pray? Have you ever considered asking that the meal itself bring Him glory? If you have felt His call to moderation at mealtime, what if you asked Him for assistance? Remember 1 Corinthians 10:31, *So, whether you eat or drink, or whatever you do, do all to the glory of God.*

Strategically filling your plate can be an act of faith, worship, and obedience. Thoughtful allocations of carbohydrates, proteins, fruits/veggies and fats determine both nutrient and calorie intake. Praying for wisdom and strength in your serving portions is an exercise in contrite surrender. Do you carefully consider your plate's composition every time you eat? Can you imagine experiencing His power perfected in your weakness at every meal? Take a moment and write a pre-consumption prayer.

The concept holds true for solo snacks and beverages, too. All offer recommended serving size, with corresponding calories. Any time you open a bag of chips, do you carefully count out a single serving, then safely tuck them back into the pantry? Most don't. We're starving, grab the bag, and devour the chips and dip until our tummy tells us we've overdone. Does it seem reasonable to pray for His fruit of self-control before opening the pantry door?

Consider the last time you opened a bag/box/barrel of some delectable goodie. Go back and honestly estimate how many servings you consumed, and how many calories that tallied. (You may need to pull the previously unopened, now empty, bag out of the trash.) Yep, size matters.

Have you ever experienced measuring your portion sizes? aka Weight Watchers. What was it like?

_____

_____

Do you have a system for determining serving sizes?

    Watch this video for tips: https://vimeo.com/48689502

Are the portions you consume when you are alone different than when you are with others? Be honest with yourself.

_____

How many times each week do you regret the amount of food you've consumed?

_____

Portion size is particularly important late in the day. As you begin to consider food as fuel vs. entertainment, like an athlete, you will eat when you need it and not when you don't. We'll dig deeper into this in our next chapter on breakfast. But what about supper? Like a marathon runner, you've crossed the finish line for the day and feel deserving of reward. Is that really when your body needs nourishment?

    Watch this video: https://vimeo.com/100749503

How do you do at eating top-heavy? Breakfast like a king, dinner like a prince, supper like a pauper. What can you do to flip your intake upside-down, from a bottom-heavy pyramid to one doing a head stand?

_____

_____

Noting plate proportions is another effective food management system, re-arranging the mid-twentieth century sections. When you consider last night's supper, what percentage of your plate did each menu item consume? i.e. How much real estate did meat nab, compared to carbs and veggies? Draw it here.

What does a healthy plate look like?

Here's the template: https://vimeo.com/45663724

What's winning your plate's territorial struggle? Meats or greens? What does Team Greens need to do to get back in the game?

_____

_____

_____

P.A.S.S.

Pray for God's transformative Spirit before every meal or snack, stirring your heart to wisdom and self-control.

Admit your tendency to overindulge.

Surrender to His Spirit. Pray during meals, especially if you find yourself eating alone. Assume Jesus is sitting in the chair next to you, encouraging wise choices.

Share this concept of dining with Jesus with someone else who struggles with portion sizes. Offer them scriptures that have helped you with trusting Him to transform your heart and your eating habits.

Fitness Focus:

1. Sane serving sizes suggest self-control, one of the fruits of the Spirit. If you find yourself struggling with over consuming, acknowledge God is the Vine and you are but a branch. Pray for His strength to calmly decline unhelpful excess. "Lord, may my portion sizes glorify You."

2. With everything you consume this week *excluding* fruits and vegetables, including beverages, note and stick to a single serving size. How does that compare with your usual consumption? What did you learn?

_____

_____

_____

3. At every meal, take the time to assess your real estate distribution. Trade some whites and browns for reds, yellows and greens.

4. Create one new recipe that includes a whole grain, lean protein, and heavy veggie.

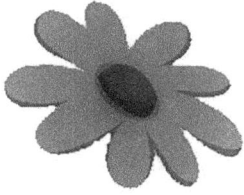

LAB 4
10:31 HABIT #2:
Fuel Early

This is the day that the LORD hath made; let us rejoice and be glad in it (Psalm 118:24).

A new day. A fresh start. Everyone knows the familiar words of wisdom. Please recite with me. "Breakfast is your . . . . . ." So why do so many skip 'cept for Starbucks?

What if you were to reframe breakfast as an act of worship. Whether you sit quietly reading His Word while savoring your coffee and eggs, or it's a rambunctious time of taming and directing kids, what better time to give thanks for all the good foods He has made for your enjoyment. Steel cut oats. Rich blueberries. An egg from a live Mama hen. It is life. It is good. It is worthy of His praise. Teach your children well to thank God for His abundant bounty.

As you are giving thanks, consider all the hands that helped get the egg from a chicken to your grocery and on to your griddle. The expanse of easily accessible foods is mind-boggling. So, while your smoothie is spinning or your veggie omelet bubbling, instead of checking Facebook, ponder the goodness of God.

"But I hate breakfast," you grumble. Remember, food is your fuel – your "go juice." A hardy start gives you the strength and vitality to think clearly and serve well. Have you ever heard yourself say, "I just don't have the energy." Then fuel up! And do you know that skipping meals teaches your body to store fat? If you're a breakfast skipper, you're surely stocking up on unwanted blubber. Aaaggg!

So . . . what is a healthy breakfast? Sugar frosted flakes? If you think so, redo Lab 2. Since we're all about eating real food, breakfast follows the same model, including those three important ingredients:

whole grain/complex carbohydrate + lean protein + fruit/veggie = great breakfast

Complex carbohydrate: Remember, you want whole, not processed, grains. Steel cut oats. Quinoa. Buckwheat. Lest we have a mutiny, we're not going to completely abandon bread, but be sure to read your labels. If the first line is "100% enriched . . ." keep seekin'. I'm a fan of Dave's Killer Bread and the Ezekiel options. (It's an acquired taste . . .)

Lean protein: Great examples are Canadian bacon or veggie sausage, peanut, almond or sunflower butter, & nuts. Then there's dairy. There are those who believe dairy is the devil, but I'd have to jump off a bridge if I was forced to give it up. You decide.

Fruit and/or veggie: We know variety is the spice of life, but many are stuck in a fruit and veggie rut, eating mostly apples and bananas, broccoli and carrots. Whattaboutamango? Ever whipped up an okra tomato sauté?

Given the formula, what breakfasts make the cut? McDonald's McGriddles? It's all about fat. Popular pastries? Where's the whole grain? Sugar pops? Hmmm.... don't think so. What is on the menu? Try some of these:

Whole wheat toast, almond butter and sliced banana or apple is my personal fav. Did you know almonds have more calcium and dietary fiber than any other nut?

Quinoa, chopped walnuts, plain Greek yogurt with a pinch of organic sugar, ground flaxseed and juicy berries.

Last night's leftovers; throw those veggies into an omelet.

Egg yolks got a bad rap in the 1990's. The character assassination was clearly without basis. Just like the ban on avocados and nuts, egg yolks slid down the drain. So sad, as the yolks are where most of the nutrients are stored. Why? 'Cuz it is the baby chick's food pantry – its primary source of nourishment. Three of many benefits of yolks include:

- strengthens your immune system
- increases eye health, including reducing risk of macular degeneration, and age-related cataracts
- improves bone density

So next time you order an egg white omelet, just know you're showing your age, following an old, outdated playbook. But make sure you're packing your personal skillet with lots of colorful veggies and a sprinkling of white vs. yellow cheese. It's lower in saturated fat.

Breakfast sandwich – This is delicious. Cook some Canadian bacon and an egg. Toast a whole wheat English muffin and fill 'er up with a tomato slice, grilled red peppers, spinach, avocado, and your favorite mustard.

Watch this video: https://vimeo.com/45794051

What's up if you are a breakfast skipper? Write your reasons here:

_____

_____

If you're busted, (You're not questioning grandma's wisdom, are you?), what do you need to do to make breakfast a habit? Be specific.

_____

_____

What breakfast options sound scrumptious to you?

_____

_____

What do you need to buy on your next trip to the market?

_____

_____

As we've discussed, simply deciding you'll start eating breakfast doesn't get it done. Transformation comes from the spirit, spurred by scripture. Meditate on the verses below, asking God to create a new heart for tending your temple in the morning.

Create in me a clean heart, O God, and renew a right spirit within me (Psalm 51:10).

I am sure of this, that he who began a good work in you will bring it to completion at the day of Jesus Christ (Philippians 1:6).

What verse will you memorize and claim this week to encourage morning feasting? Write it here.

_____

_____

How can your buddies support you?

_____

_____

Insights by Grace: https://www.livewellbygrace.com/speaking-blog/2018/6/4/scripture-spa

P.A.S.S.

Pray for a renewed enthusiasm and commitment to fueling well in the morning.

Ask for insights and ideas to make a morning meal meaningful and feasible.

Surrender to His ways and His will. If Jesus were a guest in your home, would you offer Him breakfast?

Share a new breakfast idea with a friend.

Fitness Focus:

1. Glorifying God by eating breakfast has obvious applications. Acknowledge Christ as the Bread of Life, your spiritual sustenance. Thank Him for nourishment to energize you for His service that day. And remember that a healthy breakfast fuels your brain, so you can easily recall scriptures that build you up to turn away from the pink box in the break room.

2. Consider your answers to the questions above. What thoughts about breakfast will you take off, and what will you put on?

_____

_____

_____

3. List 3 breakfasts that sound tasty to you.

_____

_____

_____

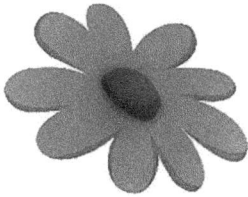

LAB 5
10:31 HABIT #3:

Color Your Plate

Oh, taste and see that the LORD is good! (Psalm 34:8)

Eat more. When was the last time your heard that? It's time to discard your can'ts and embrace the many tasty cans on your long list of real food. Relishing the plentiful bounty of multicolored fruits and veggies may be the easiest of the 10:31 Habits. When you're trying to shed some pounds and are considering the dreaded D-I-E-T, do you focus on all the scrumptious foods you have to refuse? What if instead you gave a shout out to God for all the yummy things you can and should eat? Review Appendix 1 again and ponder once more the expanse of options He has provided. The variety of tastes, textures and colors rival His floral artistry.

As we've discussed, "experts" are at odds about food guidelines. Some say high protein and no carbs. Others value whole grains but shun all animal products. Then there's the grapefruit diet . . . (Did you ever hear about Oprah's fake Hot Dog Diet?) One of the few things on which everyone seems to agree is fruits and veggies are your friends. (Well, some shun bananas and sweet potatoes . . .) Nutrient rich. High in fiber. Proven to reduce your risk of heart disease and stroke. What's not to love? The trick is including them at every feeding. Berries for breakfast. Veggies in your office snack drawer. Sandwiches with all the fixin's and lotsa color for supper. If your family is unenthusiastic, be sneaky. Load up your soups with mega veggies. Create a stir fry with a rainbow of colors. How can anyone refuse sautéed apples at supper time?*

Watch this video for some ideas: https://vimeo.com/45814261

How do you do in the produce department? Are you stuck in a rut? Iceberg lettuce and green bean casserole are the extent of your veggie adventures? When was the last time you sprinkled pomegranate seeds on your salad? Since God has been so generous, why not celebrate at every meal? Consider a platter of romantic red peppers, vibrant orange carrots, pure white cauliflower and spring green broccoli and ask yourself, "What if I had to live on manna alone?" Psalm 34:8 seems an obvious response to the variety of options God has provided. *Oh, taste and see that the LORD is good!*

---

* dice apples, cover with 1" of OJ, sprinkle with cinnamon and simmer about 20 minutes.

Kim Taylor and I did a 3-part series on *Stirring Words* entitled *Taste and See*. Here is the link to Part 1: https://www.holyhealthclub.com/new-blog/2020/8/12/taste-amp-see-part-1

Stirring Words is also available on your favorite podcast app.

Fruits and veggies are also full of fiber. If you're having trouble rallying enthusiasm for what likely feels like yet another "it's good for you" rationale, let's look at dietary fiber's function. Do you think it's solely for . . . well . . . uhh . . . you know . . . so you'll be more regular? Curing constipation is certainly a plus, but not fiber's only merit. A fiber-rich food plan also reduces your risk of Type 2 diabetes and heart disease. Interested in shedding a few pounds? Also referred to as "roughage or bulk", fiber includes all parts of plant foods that your body can't digest or absorb. (Hmmm . . . sounds sort of like the cabbage diet.) Unlike other food components like fats, proteins and carbohydrates, which your body uses for fuel, fiber isn't digested. It simply passes unchanged through your digestive system. There are two types, soluble and insoluble. The former "gets you movin'," and the latter reduces cholesterol and glucose, lowering your risk of disease.

Fiber also facilitates fat loss. Eating fiber-filled foods makes you feel full, keeping your hunger pangs at bay with fewer calories. Let me repeat that: Eating fiber-filled foods makes you feel full, keeping your hunger pangs at bay with fewer calories. So, if you're serious about weight loss, set your daily fiber fix at 25 grams.

What foods are fiber-full? Does it come in a variety of flavors like Baskin Robbins? Actually, yes! Fruits, vegetables, whole grains and legumes are the champions. Not surprising, whole vs. processed foods. Eat these for a fiber boost:

Raspberries (1/2 C) 4 gm
Orange/banana 3 gm
Blueberries (1/2 C) 2.5 gm
Pear w/skin 5 gm
Black Bean soup (1/2 C) 5 gm
Split pea soup (1/2 C) 9 gm

Ready to taste and see? Try to eat one of everything on Appendix 1 every month. Track your healthful indulgences through the rest of this study.

P.A.S.S.

Pray to have the eyes of your heart opened to new bounty-full treasures.

Ask for a colorful awakening. What luscious gifts have you been overlooking?

Surrender to His goodness. Taste and see that the Lord is good!

Share your revitalized vision of sweet treats with someone who defaults to the unhelpful. Bring them a basket of blackberries!

Fitness Focus:

1. With every different flavor you try, eat all to the glory of God. Taste and see that the Lord is good!

2. Eat one new fruit or veggie each week for the rest of this study.

3. Swap vegetarian recipes with your friends.

4. Get excited about roasted Brussels sprouts.*

5. How would you like your buddy/small group to support you? How can you encourage them?

_____

_____

_____

_____

_____

_____

---

* Roasted veggies: Chop everything up and throw in a gallon Ziplock. Don't forget onions! Add enough olive oil to sufficiently coat all the veggies. Drop your bounty on a cookie sheet and arrange into a single layer if possible, then salt if you choose. Bake at 400 degrees for 20-30 minutes, stirring often.

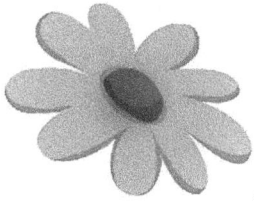

LAB 6
10:31 HABIT #4:
Shun Sugar

Turn my eyes from looking at worthless things, and give me life in Your ways (Psalm 119:37).

This is a BIG one, Church. Before stepping into this sticky topic, let's remind ourselves of Paul's twice mentioned caution: *All things are lawful, but not all things are helpful. All things are lawful, but not all things build up, . . . All things are lawful for me, but I will not be dominated by anything.* Claiming God's Word as our beacon, let's ask ourselves a few simple questions. Answer each with a 1-5 rating:

1 = absolutely not
2 = probably not
3 = don't know
4 = likely
5 = Of course!

Are sugar treats a nutritious choice?

If a brother or sister struggles with his/her weight and unhelpful food cravings, could they feel uncomfortable when presented with a table loaded with pastries?

If a Family member is diabetic or pre-diabetic, are sweets a wise choice for them? i.e. a plate of desserts taken to the shut-ins.

If a young mother with small children is being diligent at home to limit her children's consumption of sweets, do you think she feels supported in that effort when they are served cookies and cupcakes at Sunday School and VBS?

You get the point. I know I'm stirring the cookie dough here but if we are truly committed to all we do glorifying God and making choices that build one another up, does it make sense to serve sweets every time the church doors open? Can we not fellowship without sabotaging our blood sugar?

My only explanation is maybe people don't fully understand sugar's detrimental effects. "It's not good for you," isn't a strong deterrent. So, what exactly happens in your body when you consume sweets? Everything you eat is converted to glucose, your primary energy source, fueling your liver, muscles, and adipose tissue. Insulin is the hormone that moves the glucose into these cells, so the more sugar you eat the more insulin your body needs to produce to maintain balance. Until it doesn't. Take a moment to watch this informative video about how He's designed your internal fueling system to stay in check:

https://www.youtube.com/watch?v=OYH1deu7-4E&t=9s

Did that step up your awe of God a notch?

Depending on other food intake, when insulin is released into your blood stream to lower your blood sugar post-sweet, it can plunge too far. Think of the blood sugar "crash" you feel shortly after eating that piece of Dutch apple pie. Have you ever heard yourself say, "I wish I had more energy"? Then shun sugar. Another symptom of low blood sugar is blurry brain, and who needs help with that? You could even feel faint. What happens to your mood when your blood sugar goes down the drink? Let's just say, no one had better cut you off on the freeway . . .

A healthy pancreas has no problem contending with moderate sugar consumption, but sometimes it simply can't keep up with the deluge. Though it's working overtime, the insulin it's producing no longer overpowers the sweet invasion. That's called insulin resistance, which is a big step toward type 2 diabetes. If you are concerned, get a fasting blood sugar test. I highly recommend WalkInLab.com. Just go to their website, search for fasting blood glucose, choose Lab Corp or Quest, find your local lab, pay and go. So simple, and your results will land in your email a few days later. https://www.walkinlab.com/

In addition to converting sugar into energy, insulin also stimulates the storage of fat, so the more sugar you eat, the more insulin you produce, and the more likely you will increase your body fat percentage. (You no longer look at total weight, right?) Along with obesity and tooth decay, sugar has also been linked to more serious health conditions, including increased mood swings (depression), a debilitated immune system and as mentioned above, adult onset diabetes.

It seems a bit dramatic to talk about addiction in reference to food, doesn't it? But consider some of the research. It's been clearly proven that sugar activates the brain's pleasure center. Surprise, surprise. We don't eat Ding Dongs under duress. Unfortunately, happy brain produces chemicals that make you want more – crave more. In fact, those chemicals are the same as those produced in heroin and morphine users. A study showed just the sight of an ice cream cone generated the same stimulation of pleasure in the brain as images of crack pipes did for addicts. What does that tell us? Sugar is addictive. The more you eat the more you want. Give kids (and big kids) cupcakes at church and they'll be internally programmed to want more the rest of the day.

Here is a terrific explanation of sugar's effects on our brain and behavior:

https://youtu.be/lEXBxijQREo

You might be saying to yourself, "I don't eat that much sugar." Is that true? Take this survey: https://www.doctoroz.com/quiz/quiz-are-you-addicted-sugar

What did you learn?

_____

_____

Where/when do you over-consume sugar?

_____

_____

What specific, small changes can you make to reduce your intake?

_____

_____

How can your friend/small group support you?

_____

_____

P.A.S.S.

Pray for the hedge of the Holy Spirit to protect you from the devil's lies that you need something sweet.

Ask him to hold your hand every time you enter a situation rife with sweet temptation. Beseech Him to remove the allure, and open your heart to the joy of temple care.

Surrender to His strength, for it is your only hope. Like the Israelites with their back against the Red Sea with Pharaoh's army upon them, He will fight the battle for His glory.

Share your sincere gratitude for a God whose love is unwavering. Tell everyone who will listen that He is faithful to those who trust in Him. The more you give God the glory, the more victories will be won.

Fitness Focus:

1. Pray Paul's admonitions in 1 Corinthians. "Lord, though through Your grace all things are lawful for me, give me the wisdom and strength to choose only what is helpful and builds me and others up. Father, show me where I am dominated by certain foods, and in the name of my Lord and Savior, Jesus, I pray you break that stronghold."

2. What verse(s) will you claim for strength when you are feeling tempted to indulge?

   _____

   _____

3. How can you contribute to the church's food fellowship offerings so you know you'll have something satisfying to eat?

   _____

   _____

4. Who in your church family also struggles with overeating sugar? How will the two of you uplift one another?

   _____

   _____

Let's see what Miss Grace has to say:
https://www.livewellbygrace.com/speaking-blog/2018/10/16/sugar-love

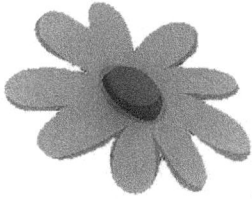

LAB 7
10:31 HABIT #5:
STOP! Eating

His delight is in the law of the LORD and in His law he mediates day and night (Psalm 1:2).

Evening eating is detrimental; gauge your feelings the morning after.

How much do you typically consume post-supper? Remember the wisdom of Kenny Rogers? "You've got to know when to hold 'em, know when to fold 'em, know when to walk away, and know when to *run*." Sing that after supper, folks. In your quiet (aka bored, lonely), evening time, when the fridge keeps calling your name, run from temptation. Lock it, along with the pantry doors. (Though surely no enticements remain in your prepared pantry.) Consider a consumption curfew.

Watch this video: https://vimeo.com/100432550

Remember Paul's instruction to take off the old, and put on the new? And Thomas Chalmers' thoughtful treatise which said, "The heart must have something to cling to – and never by its own voluntary consent will it so denude itself of all its attachments." (p. xx) Never in your own strength will you be able to snub the irksome hounding to nibble at night. Only by clinging to something else, God and His Word, will you successfully silence Satan's coaxing.

When people think about improving their food, they mostly consider content. More veggies, less pizza. But the truth is, timing of your meals matters as much as what you choose to chew. We discussed the importance of starting your days with breakfast. You've got that nailed, right? But your body's need for fuel late in the day is minimal. How many calories do you need to watch a movie? So, after your light supper, STOP eating, specifically, at least three hours before bedtime. In fact, I'd recommend a 12-hour fast. i.e. 6pm-6am. Why? First, because if you have fueled well all day, you don't need to eat. Second, because typically evening snacking isn't stellar sustenance. Do you really crave carrots at night? Finally, and most importantly, especially if late-night eating is a stronghold, it's an exercise in dependency on your Source. Instead of snacking, sip herb tea and sup on the Word. He will cure you of cravings.

Let's look at this from our 1 Corinthians 10:31 perspective. If your behavior change goal is to depend upon God and give Him glory, what if you accepted his offer to strap on His yoke after supper. If evening eating has always been a pothole for you, do something drastic. Fast.

Fasting is a dying discipline. Like the Bornean orangutan, it's on the endangered species list. In fact, fasting may group you with the fanatics. But Jesus was known for slipping into the wilderness to pray and feast solely on God's presence. If you're not quite ready to live on chicken broth for forty days, what if you began by shunning all food for the three hours before you go to bed? Given that's a time of high temptation, it's the perfect opportunity to take off the desires of the flesh and put on the redeeming Word of God.

Miss Grace has an idea to help you shun the Devil's late-night bait: https://www.livewellbygrace.com/speaking-blog/2019/6/3/evening-feasting

How do you do? If you're nighty-night by 10 p.m., do you quit eating by 7? Back in the day when Oprah was training with Bob Greene, she said, "He won't even let me eat one grape after 7 p.m.!" Does your consumption exceed a solo grape?

P.A.S.S.

Pray for spiritual healing over the stronghold of evening eating.

Ask for God's help in redirecting your thoughts to praise and trust Him.

Surrender to His strength. You absolutely cannot stop in your own power.

Share your story with someone else. Pray and read the Word with a buddy or two. Create an evening eating hotline for your church family. This could be a sensational outreach ministry! Do you know how many people eat in the evenings out of loneliness?

Fitness Focus:

1. Declare evening hours a time of fasting, depending on Him and Him alone for strength in refraining from unhelpful eating and dominating cravings. Choose a verse(s) to meditate upon and memorize, acknowledging God as your only sustenance.

2. Review your redefined Why from the first chapter. Are you keeping your eyes on that prize? Maybe it's time to post it on the refrigerator so it shouts at you late at night.

3. Make a pact with your pal and/or small group to STOP! eating three hours before bedtime, and to call for help if you're ready to falter. Like an A.A. sponsor, be prepared to pull your buddy off a craving cliff.

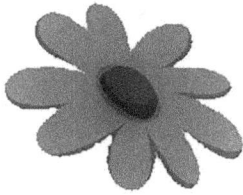

LAB 8
10:31 HABIT #6:

MOVE! *Often*

Let them praise His name with dancing (Psalm 149:3).

You knew this one was coming. But now that all that you do is for the glory of God, walking has been grace-fully transformed into Worship Workouts™. (Reread *Revere His Greatness*, p. 89) You're ready to get up and *GO!* Right?

You've heard the wisdom of unidentified experts chiding "Exercise is good for you," but it isn't getting you off the couch. With this new view of it being an uplifting opportunity for praise, will your interest increase? Let's peer into your noggin for a moment: What words/phrases/images historically come to mind when you consider exercise? Be honest.

In the space below, list both the benefits and drawbacks of exercise. Again, be candid. Note everything that for you is a positive result of being active, and what is the downside.

If you are like most people, the plusses outweigh the minuses, which confirms your sedentary tendencies aren't because of a perceived lack of benefit. It's more about . . . . what? What keeps you from getting going? Remember, honesty (with yourself) is the best policy.

Ready to get started? Not quite? Need a little more inspiration? Consider this: How would you like to be smarter? Better able to remember and stay focused? Reduce your risk of dementia and Alzheimer's disease?

Watch this video: https://www.ted.com/talks/wendy_suzuki_the_brain_changing_benefits_of_exercise?utm_source=tedcomshare&utm_medium=email&utm_campaign=tedspread#t-543118

As busy as you are it's easy to say, "I just don't have time . . . ," but exercise is imperative, gang. Temple maintenance requires *moving* daily.

At the end of the video above, Dr. Suzuki led her audience in one minute of movement. Her chants were self-affirming. Instead, what if you used your walk time to memorize scripture? Your body is flooded with oxygen so there's no better time to engrain the Word into your brain. Move and memorize!

If we're going to make a dent in doing life differently, let's start with some paralysis analysis: Why types of exercise do you enjoy? (Now come on, you can't tell me you detest every activity except walking the mall . . .)

Look at your life and your days. Is there any small slot in your schedule to sneak in a walk? Important note: If a 30-minute window is nowhere to be found, two fifteens are great.

What hurdles (aka: excuses) have you encountered in the past that kept you stuck in your sluggishness? How do you intend to overcome them this time? What scriptures will you claim when temptation is trying to topple you? Remember, there are several in the previous pages.

One of the easiest ways to sustain your commitment to move regularly is to make it fun. I heard a story years ago about a gal who was having a tough time staying committed to riding her exercise bike. Then I learned it was down in a cold, dank basement! Really? That is reminiscent of what we think a life following Christ might be like – difficult and boring. But *we* make it that way! The only criteria for moving is . . . *moving!* So, stand up and dance!

https://vimeo.com/115614361

List 3 other ways you can make exercise fun:

1. _____

2. _____

3. _____

Exercise Intensity

Your heart is a muscle, and you want it to be stronger, right? Then you need to work it beyond what it is accustomed. Just like wielding dumbbells builds your biceps, your heart gets stronger when you regularly rev it up. We call this exercise intensity. On a scale of 1-10, how hard are you pushing yourself on that exercise bike? If it's below 5, you're riding for recreation, which is a great way to reduce stress. If you deem your ride a 5-6, that's a perfect fat-burning rate. It's when you begin to huff and puff, scoring the effort a 7-8, that you're toughening your ticker.

Watch this video: https://vimeo.com/48807580

IMPORTANT: READ THIS

If you are just getting started on an exercise program, have a heart condition, and/or are overweight, *start out slowly*, keeping your heart rate below 120bpm (beats per minute). As your physical condition improves you can push a little harder. This is why we recommend using a heart monitor.

There's an App for That.

We live by our phones, literally and figuratively. So yes, there's lots to discover in the mobile health/fitness world. Check out MyFitnessPal and TrackMyRun. There are several yoga apps, and don't miss Christian Fitness TV and Revelation Wellness on YouTube.

P.A.S.S.

Pray for divine inspiration to move often and intently, and for ways to enjoy His presence with you.

Ask for God to make you sorely uncomfortable in the spirit any time you are considering punting. (Are you really ready to ask that?)

Surrender to this sometimes inconvenient discipline, knowing it is good for you both physically and spiritually. You are out there in His strength!

Share His love by inviting someone to hike or attend an exercise class with you. Start a weekly walk from your church, encouraging everyone to invite an unsaved friend.

Fitness Focus:

1. In every walk or bike ride you take, do all to the glory of God. Imagine Him with you, thrilled with your renewed commitment to care for the temple of the Holy Spirit. Oh, the joy of pleasing our Father!

2. For the next four weeks, to what days, time, activity, and intensity can you realistically commit?

   _____

   _____

3. Share your intention with your buddy or small group.

4. What supportive scripture(s) will you memorize?

_____

_____

5. When you are on the verge of bailing out, take an honest assessment. In that moment, what functional god are you worshipping? (ouch . . .)

6. Determine how/who you will support in their active commitment.

_____

_____

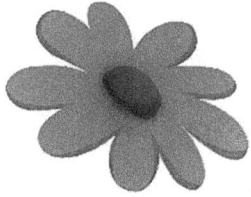

LAB 9
10:31 HABIT #7:
Strength Training

The joy of the Lord is your strength (Nehemiah 8:10).

Enjoying the Lord brings strength, and so does resistance training.

Building muscle is a miracle. What a wonder to pump baby dumbbells while you walk and watch your biceps bulge. Give God glory for this gracious gift!

Jesus was clear that we are no longer in bondage to sin. John 8:36 tells us that if Jesus sets you free, you are *free indeed*. Undeniably free. Strength training can be an awe-inspiring example of our freedom. You are not destined to frailty and feebleness. You are not irreversibility condemned to falls and fractures. Instead, by the miracle of muscle development, you can experience the liberty of physical strength for all of your days. Rejoice!

"Use 'em or lose 'em." You're familiar with the phrase, but like the breakfast mantra, it blows through your brain and floats away. Let me tell you sisters, frail went out of style in the 50's. You don't need to be an athletic animal, but wouldn't it be great to be able to carry your groceries without grimacing, or pull the trash cans to the curb without calling for hubby to help? (Oh . . . sorry . . . that's a boy job.) The only thing that keeps you from beefy biceps is baby dumbbells. No, you don't need to go to a gym and press a 50-pound barbell. A 1-2 pound weight will rock your upper body.

Watch this video: https://vimeo.com/92798721

Don't you love multi-tasking? Walk with mini-weights and you'll strengthen your upper body *and* your heart by pushing your pulse higher, *and* burn more calories! What's not to love?

If there's anyone out there not yet convinced (no worries, I've worked with skeptics before . . .), here's another bennie of resistance training: it builds bone density. Remember our DXA scan discussion in the Fitness Figures section? Women's bones start deteriorating about the age of 30. Any 30+ers in the crowd? Then guess what, your bones are slowly disintegrating. Seriously. Over time they start to resemble Swiss cheese. (And you thought wrinkles were a problem.) Then guess what happens when you're older and your balance begins to fail? You fall and break something. But that doesn't need to happen. Walking strengthens both muscles and bone, upper and lower body, because remember, you're walking with weights!

Need some more ideas for muscle maintenance?

Watch these videos:

Love Those Lunges https://vimeo.com/48764047

Abs-olutely https://vimeo.com/38377379

Marine Workout https://vimeo.com/48691071

Let Lt. Col. Tom show you some tricks on the fitness ball:

Ball Intro https://vimeo.com/79564529

Push-ups https://vimeo.com/80752991

Flies https://vimeo.com/84446784

Core https://vimeo.com/91578303

P.A.S.S.

Pray through the idea that spiritual and physical strength build each other up. "Lord, through Your strength I can build my strength."

Ask God to open your eyes to the many opportunities for minutes for strength training.

Surrender your resistant thoughts about resistance training. Renew your mind with a vision of yourself strong and sturdy.

Share what you've learned about the benefits of strength training with someone else. Buy them a ball, mat, and baby dumbbells.

Fitness Focus:

1. Celebrate the miracle of muscle building! As you walk with weights, do your ball exercises, and/or squat while you're prepping supper, do all for God's glory!

2. Have a handful of scriptures printed and handy in your pocket to preach to yourself when you're considering bailing out on your strength training session.

3. Talk to your buddy and/or small group about why in the world you wouldn't walk with weights.

4. What mutual commitment to accountability will ya'll make? Accountable to what exactly? When? Where? For how long? Be specific!

_____

_____

_____

_____

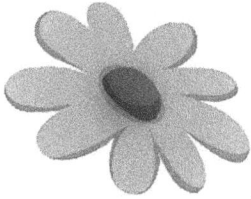

LAB 10
10:31 HABIT #8:
S-T-R-E-T-C-H

You keep him in perfect peace whose mind is stayed on You, because he trusts in You (Isaiah 26:3).

Faith brings perfect peace.

Much has been said about control, idols, pride, faith vs. fickle feelings. Stretching can become a physical manifestation of spiritual surrender. Take a deep breath, and let go.

For most, stretching is another should. You're sure it would reduce your shoulder, neck, and/or back pain. You know you shouldn't sit so long at your computer. And taking time to breathe and stretch deeply would be wonderfully relaxing.

But you don't.

Why not?

It's tough to blame it on lack of time because much can be made of a minute. More likely, you simply don't think about it. You're programmed to brush your teeth before bed, but not to lie on the floor to stretch your back. Is there a way to tie the two together?

As we discussed in Re-defining Your Why, we tend to those things that bring the most reward. You go to work so you can pay the bills and buy nice things. You do a *lot* for your family because you love loving on them. Have you ever considered the ROI (return on investment) of stretching? Write your perceived benefits here:

_____

_____

_____

If the above space is blank, allow me:

1. Increased flexibility – But . . . so what? To minimize pain. To reduce your risk of injury. "But I'm not out on the field/court anymore," you might be saying. But do you ever lift anything heavy? Have you had to sprint after a wayward child? Stand on your tippy-toes and reach for something on a high shelf? If your

muscles are tight, you are risking injury. (Maybe that new pain in your back will help you remember to stretch before bed . . .)

2. Improved circulation – Many suffer from blurry brain mid-morning and/or mid-afternoon. If that includes you, stand up and stretch. It will stimulate both your circulation and mental juices.
3. Improved balance – The more flexible you are, the more balanced you'll be. As you age you have a higher risk of falling, but it is reduced if you maintain your strength and flexibility. (Old . . . me?)

But maybe most importantly, stretching is stress management. Oh sure, it's great to go to Hawaii and sit on the beach for a week, but what about the other fifty-one? Any time you're starting to sizzle, go to a quiet place, take several deep breaths and stretch. Blood pressure and tension will dwindle.

The coolest thing about stretching is it can be done just about anywhere, any time, and seriously, seconds can give your body a hug. Consider these scenarios:

You're standing in line at the grocery store and you're tempted to be tempted by the candy bars. Instead, stand at a 45-degree angle to your cart, with your shoulder to the push handle. Turn to hold the handle with both hands. Using the cart for stability, gently twist forward to stretch your back. Breathe deeply. Switch sides.

You're sitting on the sidelines at your kid's soccer game. Cross one ankle over the opposite knee. Sit up tall, keep your torso straight (don't arch your back), head high, and slowly bend forward. It won't take much movement before you feel an ouch in your bum. Switch sides.

While you're sitting there, extend one leg at a 45-degree angle, toe pointed up. Like before, keep your torso tall and slowly bend forward. Feel your hamstring howl? Switch sides.

Here's the point. Stretching doesn't take a ton of time; it just entails intention. But a few words of caution:

✓ Never bounce or push. Stretching should be relaxing, not painful. Oh, you might feel a little squeak, but don't push into pain.
✓ Ideally, hold each stretch for 30 seconds.
✓ Breathe. Literally, think about pushing oxygen into that muscle. (Go ahead, I dare you. Talk to it.)

√ Relax. Let go. Pray. Stretching, for me, is a sweet time with my Father. It is a quiet moment of listening. As I feel my muscles releasing, I envision my heart also surrendering to His Spirit. Stretch with an anticipation of both physical and spiritual surrender.

P.A.S.S.

Pray to better surrender to His way and His will, and that He would nudge you to see moments when you can stop, breathe, stretch, and better surrender.

Ask God to speak to you when you are surrendered and stretching. Oh the things He might reveal when we slow down to listen!

Surrender to whatever He whispers to you in your stretching time.

Share your stretching sessions, even if its virtually. While you're chatting with your bestie, why wouldn't you use your Bluetooth and be on your mat stretching? (Or in the soft, green grass – aaahhhh.)

Fitness Focus:

1. We glorify God by our full-hearted faith in Him. As you breathe into a relaxing stretch, surrender all your fears, concerns, and complaints to your Father.

2. Think about when you can add quiet moments into your busy day to stretch. Be specific about time and place.

3. Take out your 10:31 Habits log and add stretching to your weekly tally.

4. Is your buddy or small group ready to commit to regular stretching? What if you did it together while talking on the phone? Or before Bible study started? Who will lead?

_____

_____

_____

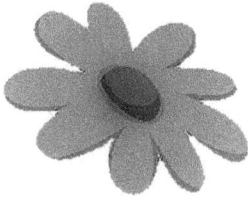

10:31 HABIT #9:
Drink Up

. . . whoever drinks of the water that I will give him will never be thirsty again (John 4:13).

Jesus got thirsty. He walked many miles on hot days, and needed to stay hydrated. While passing through Samaria, "enemy territory," He asked a woman to draw Him a drink from the well. *How is it that you, a Jew, ask for a drink from me, a woman of Samaria?* (John 4:9) He was breaking all the rules. But per usual, he used the analogy of a physical need to present a spiritual truth. He referred to true faith in Him as *living water.* What if with every sip throughout every day we gave glory to God as the only One who can truly quench our thirst?

Have you ever been thirsty? *Really* thirsty? What's the one and only thing you think about? Water. Not a cheeseburger. Not chicken nachos. Water. Plain ol' thirst quenching water. Most everyone has heard the recommendation to drink 64 oz. of water a day, but it's another one of those suggestions we too often ignore. But actually, it's sort of a big deal because your body is about 65% water, and your brain 85%! As little as 2% water loss begins to impact your brain function and you'll start to feel fatigued, because your metabolism is slowing down. So, if fuzzy brain isn't enough to motivate you to drink your 64, a sluggish engine that burns fewer calories may motivate you.

Keeping sufficiently hydrated is particularly important for seniors. Many worry about getting dementia or worse. They start to get a little teettery, and that's unnerving. They also may not have the energy they used to. This combination of conditions can create anxiety. But what if they're simply dehydrated, and could feel stronger, sharper and more stable by drinking more fluids?

Here are a few fun facts: You lose about 8 to 10 cups of water per normal day through breathing, sweating, and basic body movements. When the sun is shining and the mercury rises, you need even more water. If you're working or playing outside on a hot day you can lose about two pounds of water per *hour.* Sweating is your personal air conditioning system, but it obviously extracts water. Like your house cleaning habits, your thirst meter lags behind your actual need, so by the time you feel thirsty your body is unhappy. Drink up early. This is especially true for exercisers. Aim for three cups of water several hours before heading out. Down another two cups 10 to 15 minutes before and keep drinking during your workout. You'll need about 4-8 oz. every 15 to 30 minutes, depending upon your intensity and weather conditions. If you don't drink enough you will be at a performance disadvantage (If you're like me, you don't need any additional handicaps . . .), and you may experience headache and/or fatigue. Have you ever seen someone weigh themselves after exercise and say, "Oh goody! Two pounds." Don't do the happy dance yet; it was just water. Drink two cups of fluid for each pound lost.

Doctors now believe a whopping 75% of us may be running around dehydrated. And take note:

- 2-5% percent dehydration is enough to influence your reaction times, which impacts your personal safety.
- 6-10% is "cause for immediate concern," warn the experts.
- 11-15% is severe, and you'll likely land in the hospital with intravenous injections.
- Over 15% can end in death.

How do you know if you're dehydrated? Thirst can actually be mistaken for hunger. (And who wouldn't rather eat a candy bar than drink a glass of water . . .) We usually don't even feel thirsty until we're moderately dehydrated, which remember was called "cause for immediate concern." By that time, you're already not thinking clearly and don't even realize it.

So be on the alert for other symptoms of dehydration:

- Your lips or mouth feel dry.
- Your heart rate and breathing increases.
- Your blood pressure may drop, so you feel unbalanced, dizzy or fatigued.
- Maybe you get a headache that won't go away, a stomach ache, or experience low back pain.
- Begin to become mentally irritated and depressed.
- And obviously your urine output diminishes.

You can see how easy it is for dehydration to go mis-diagnosed. For more on the importance of hydrating, especially if you are "gracefully seasoned."

Watch this video: https://vimeo.com/97749489

The good news is it's super simple to stay hydrated. A person who requires 2000 calories per day needs about 6 to 8 cups of liquids. Water, especially chilled, makes a beeline from your digestive tract to your tissues and cools you inside and out. Plain water is best but you'll be thrilled to know coffee and tea work too. Water also comes from food sources. Fruits, vegetables, and even meats and cheeses are full of H2O.

▶ Watch this video: https://vimeo.com/97182058

Here are some other ideas:

- Always keep a water bottle or large glass close by, sipping it constantly.
- Add flavor with lemon or herb tea to make it more palatable.
- Drink carbonated water & lime for a different twist.
- Drink a glass of water immediately in the morning and at every meal.
- Help your hydration by eating lots of fruits & veggies which have a high water content.

Remember that alcohol dehydrates you, so chase your cocktail with some agua.

Back to Jesus and the Samaritan woman. He said to her, *everyone who drinks of this water will be thirsty again, but whoever drinks of the water that I will give him will never be thirsty again. The water that I will give him will become in him a spring of water welling up to eternal life* (John 4:13-14). In the spiritual realm, God and His Word are our fountain of life. Read Psalm 42:1-2. Do you pant for God like a thirsty deer?

Why do you think Jesus chose the analogy of thirst? Does this reinforce the idea of Him being our fount? Why or why not?

_____

_____

_____

P.A.S.S.

Pray for those who have no clean water to drink, and lift your voice in genuine thanksgiving that it is so easily accessible for us. We are indeed blessed.

Ask God to nudge you to drink often. Choose eight different people you want to pray for each day, and lift them up to the Lord as you drink the glass in their honor.

Surrender your stubborn heart if you hear yourself saying, "I hate to drink water!" Think instead of replenishing the liquids your body needs for a sharp mind and robust energy.

Share hydration hints with your friends. i.e. add lemon or cucumber to your water, drink 1:4 bubbly water and OJ or cranberry juice, savor herb tea.

Fitness Focus:

1. Drink generously, acknowledging grand gratitude for your Living Water.

2. Add water to your 10:31 Habit list and start tracking it this week.

3. Buy yourself a fun bottle or mug (or both) so your beverage is handy.

4. Have a friend who needs to drink more water? Buy her a bottle too.

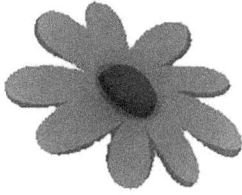

LAB 12
10:31 HABIT #10:

Rest

Come to Me, all who are weary and heavy-laden, and I will give you rest
(Matthew 11:28, NASB).

Rest requires faith. We do and do because we believe we must. We rely on our own efforts for the results we want. That wasn't God's message to the people of Judah in 2 Chronicles. Jehoshaphat was surrounded by three threatening armies. He bowed before God, fessed up to his fear and powerlessness, but declared, *We do not know what to do, but our eyes are on you.* God immediately replied, "I've got this." *Stand firm. Hold your position. The battle is not yours, but God's* (2 Chronicles 20:17).

Have you ever been in a situation where God said, "Sit still. Rest. Let me handle this." But you didn't. You kept meddling, thinking God needed your help. Isaiah 30:15 reads, *In returning and rest you shall be saved; in quietness and in trust shall be your strength.* Oh, so counter-intuitive to our culture!

Rest throughout our days also requires trust in provision beyond our own making. Are you working 50-60 hour weeks, believing you must to make ends meet? Are you cherishing Sundays for Sabbath rest?

Many (most) of us are uncomfortable resting. It feels unproductive. Time-wasting. Sluggardly. But like it or not, God calls us to slow down. To be still. He speaks often about His call to Sabbath rest, intricately entwined with resting in His steadfast love and faithfulness. Read and reflect on the scriptures below, noting the whisper of His Spirit:

> Deuteronomy 5:14
> Jeremiah 31:2-3, 25
> Matthew 11:29

How do you do in recognizing and honoring the Sabbath? Is it normally a peaceful, replenishing day for you?

_____

_____

_____

What sabotages your relaxation on Sundays? How can you change that?

_____

_____

_____

Do you take time during your busy days for short breaks? Why or why not? Would you like to change that? Be specific. i.e. I will sit at 3:00 p.m. every day and read my Bible for 15 minutes.

Though it's important to schedule uncommitted, peaceful time to relax and rejuvenate, you needn't panic. It doesn't have to take hours and hours. In fact, you can reduce your heart rate, blood pressure, and stress in minutes. Want to know how?

Watch this video: https://vimeo.com/78087647

Take a moment, right now, to put aside your electronic device, adjust yourself so you're sitting comfortably, close your eyes, roll your shoulders a bit, and do some deep breathing.

It's not a surprise that walking in the wild has proven to reduce blood pressure, anxiety and stress. When was the last time you walked in the woods?

Watch this video: https://vimeo.com/114518537

Not only have Christians, like the world, created chaotic lives, many are also sleep deprived. And the scary truth is so are our children. Dr. Cindy Gellner says, "for kids between the ages of 6 and 19, 41% who had their mobile device in the bedroom didn't sleep enough hours." [https://healthcare.utah.edu/the-scope/shows.php?shows=0_hsegy53m] Kids are futzing with their phones, being stimulated by both the light and the content, so they don't nod off until the wee hours. But nightly rest, 7-8 hours minimum, is one of the required habits for health. Let's flip to an Old Testament story when one of God's own was exhausted. Remember Elijah's brazenness, daring the gods of Baal to start a bonfire? And when they couldn't he had them douse the wood pile with water and his God started the weenie roast? Do you also remember Queen Jezebel, Ahab's wife, wasn't very happy over the humiliation? She threatened to kill Elijah, so he ran for his life. When he finally crumbled under a broom tree he started whining to God. "Father, I'm over this harsh world! That crazy woman is scary! I'm ready to die..." Ever feel down and defeated by the challenges of this world? As we read on, what did Elijah do? (1 Kings 19)

Yep. He slept. ZZzzz . . . . Snoozin' under a shade tree. Think there's a message here?

A whole slew of Americans are running around sleep deprived, which impacts us all in small and significant ways. Employees are less productive. Colleagues are cranky. And fatigued drivers can cause havoc and horror on the road.

Like most things, setting yourself up for a good night's sleep requires some strategy. How do you do?

Watch this video: https://vimeo.com/128092248

Do you regularly get seven or more hours of sleep each night? If not, what evening habits are stirring up your spirit?

_____

_____

How can you stage yourself for deep sleep?

_____

_____

Looking for a Good Book? Here's a hint: *This book of the law shall not depart from your mouth, but you shall meditate on it day and night . . . For then you will make your way prosperous, and then you will have good success* (Joshua 1:8).

If someone shares your bed, can you make a healthy sleep pact?

_____

_____

P.A.S.S.

Pray for God's wisdom and direction on rest. Where are you doing vs. believing? In what area has He told you to stand firm and be quiet, allowing Him to manage the battle?

Ask for faith to rest.

Surrender yourself, your time, your fears. Tell Him why it's scary to slow down.

Share your journey with a friend who's also always on the go. Maybe you can both start with the small step of stretch (10:31 #8) and rest.

Fitness Focus:

1. Memorize Isaiah 30:15.

2. Give thanks to God for the gift of rest, and embrace it in faith, which gives him glory.

3. Assess your before-bed habits. What do you need to tweak? Who will you ask to hold you accountable?

4. Commit to taking 5 minutes every day this week to sit still and breathe deeply. Whisper scripture if you please.

6. Call up a friend you haven't seen for a while and schedule a wilderness walk. For you city folks, that could be a local park.

Final Thought

As I envision people completing this process – eating more healthfully, moving more regularly, and most importantly, surrendering more fully, I am encouraged. As you might imagine, the corporate wellness world left me unfulfilled. Oh, sure, people changed their behavior in spurts, embracing the designated healthy habits long enough to complete a fitness challenge. But soon after winning the t-shirt, they'd revert right back to their well-entrenched ways. External rewards rarely work.

Romans 5 reminds us that suffering produces endurance, character, and hope, and *hope does not disappoint, because the love of God has been poured out within our hearts through the Holy Spirit who was given to us* (Romans 5:5). So, rejoice, saints. Again I say, rejoice! You are a new creation. Through Christ, you can live fully and abundantly. You may not yet be the perfect eater or most rigorous exerciser, but remember Tricia's counsel: "A slip-up isn't a relapse." Your stony heart is slowly being softened as it submits to the Spirit. For as you behold the glory of the Lord, *you are being transformed into the same image from one degree of glory to another. For this comes from the Lord who is the Spirit* (2 Corinthians 3:18).

Claim it, Church.

APPENDIX 1:
Fruit & Veggie List

Have you had your 9 today??

Apple	Currants	Pear
Apricot	Dates	Peas
Artichoke	Eggplant	Peppers
Arugula	Fig	Pineapple
Asparagus	Grapefruit	Plums
Avocado	Grapes	Pomegranate
Banana	Green Beans	Potato
Beets	Greens	Prunes
Blackberries	(collards, turnip, dandelion, mustard)	Pumpkin
Blueberries	Jicama	Radish
Bok Choy	Kale	Raisins
Boysenberries	Kiwi	Raspberries
Broccoli	Kumquat	Rutabaga
Brussels sprouts	Leek	Spinach
Cabbage	Lemon	Squash
Cantaloupe	Lime	Strawberries
Carrot	Mango	Sweet potato / yam
Cauliflower	Melon (cantaloupe, honeydew)	Tangerine
Celery	Nectarine	Tomato
Cherries	Okra	Turnip
Corn	Orange	Watercress
Cranberries	Papaya	Zucchini
Cucumber	Peach	

Royalty Reminders

O LORD, you have searched me and known me!
²You know when I sit down and when I rise up;
you discern my thoughts from afar.
³You search out my path and my lying down
and are acquainted with all my ways.
⁴Even before a word is on my tongue,
behold, O Lord, you know it altogether.
⁵You hem me in, behind and before,
and lay your hand upon me.
⁶Such knowledge is too wonderful for me;
it is high; I cannot attain it (Psalm 139:1-6).

For if while we were enemies we were reconciled to God by the death of his Son, much more, now that we are reconciled, shall we be saved by his life (Romans 5:10).

¹⁵For you did not receive the spirit of slavery to fall back into fear, but you have received the Spirit of adoption as sons, by whom we cry, "Abba! Father!" ¹⁶The Spirit himself bears witness with our spirit that we are children of God, ¹⁷and if children, then heirs— heirs of God and fellow heirs with Christ, provided we suffer with him in order that we may also be glorified with him (Romans 8:15-17).

⁹But you are a chosen race, a royal priesthood, a holy nation, a people for his own possession, that you may proclaim the excellencies of him who called you out of darkness into his marvelous light. ¹⁰Once you were not a people, but now you are God's people; once you had not received mercy, but now you have received mercy (I Peter 2:9-10).

¹¹In him we have obtained an inheritance, having been predestined according to the purpose of him who works all things according to the counsel of his will, ¹²so that we who were the first to hope in Christ might be to the praise of his glory. ¹³In him you also, when you heard the word of truth, the gospel of your salvation, and believed in him, were sealed with the promised Holy Spirit, ¹⁴who is the guarantee of our inheritance until we acquire possession of it, to the praise of his glory (Ephesians 1:11-14).

APPENDIX 3:
Sample Shopping List

Fruits/Veggies: The more the healthier! Including bags of spinach, arugula, yams, . . .

Meats/protein:
Chicken
Fish
Extra lean ground beef or turkey
Hummus
Nuts – almonds, walnuts, pecans
Almond/peanut butter

Whole Grains:
Brown rice
Wild rice
Quinoa
Old Fashioned Oatmeal
Wheat berries

BE ADVENTURESOME!
Buy a new grain every month give it a try.

Dairy:
Nonfat/low fat milk
Lowfat cottage cheese
Lowfat cheese
Lowfat yogurt – vanilla and/or plain
Greek yogurt
Light cream cheese
Eggs

Canned goods:
Variety of beans
Tomato sauce & tomatoes
Sugar free pineapple
Peas
Corn

Condiments:
Fun mustards
Salsa
Ketchup
BBQ sauce
Low Sodium Teriyaki sauce
Low Sodium Soy sauce

APPENDIX 4:

Fitness Record

FITNESS RECORD FOR: _____

	Goal Weight	Actual Weight	Goal BC	Actual BC	Goal B.P.	Actual B.P.	Goal RHR	Actual RHR	Goal RR	Actual RR	Goal VO2	Actual VO2	Goal Chol.	Actual Chol.	Goal Risk Ratio	Actual Risk Ratio	Goal Push Ups	Actual Push Ups	Goal Sit Ups	Actual Sit Ups	Goal Set-Reach	Actual Set-Reach
January																						
February																						
March																						
April																						
May																						
June																						
July																						
August																						
September																						
October																						
November																						
December																						

Fitness Record Key: Weight Optional, B.C. = Body Composition, B.P. = Blood Pressure,
RHR = Resting Heart Rate, RR = Recovery Rate, VO2 = Aerobic Capacity, Chol. = Cholesterol

Weekly Reckoning

Spiraling toward sanctification requires regular reckoning – reviewing, assessing and correcting your choices. Like any other aspiration or goal, progress must be regularly reevaluated to stay on course. Take some quiet time each week with your Guide, talking over the trek.

Spiritual Disciplines:

What has God asked of me spiritually?

How have I responded?

What is my next right step?

What scripture(s) will I claim to strengthen my spiritual resolve?

How can my friend help encourage me?

Who and how can I encourage someone spiritually this week?

Physical Disciplines:

What has God asked of me physically?

How have I responded?

What is my next right step?

What scripture(s) will I claim to strengthen my physical resolve?

How can my friend help encourage me?

Who and how can I encourage someone physically this week?

APPENDIX 6:

Recommended Reading

Seeing With New Eyes, David Powlison

Instruments in the Redeemers Hands, Paul David Tripp

How People Change, Paul Tripp & Timothy Lane

Respectable Sins, Jerry Bridges

O. Hallesby's book on prayer

Fresh Wind, Fresh Fire by Jim Cymbala

Several classic works can nurture your spiritual disciplines. *Celebration of Discipline*, by Richard Foster.*The Spirit of the Disciplines*, by Dallas Willard, and the incomparable work, *Knowing God*, by J.I. Packer. Listen to this Piper podcast to set the stage for the purpose of spiritual disciplines: https://www.desiringgod.org/interviews/what-are-spiritual-disciplines

www.ingramcontent.com/pod-product-compliance
Lightning Source LLC
Chambersburg PA
CBHW080358030426
42334CB00024B/2915